THE COMPLETE GUIDE TO

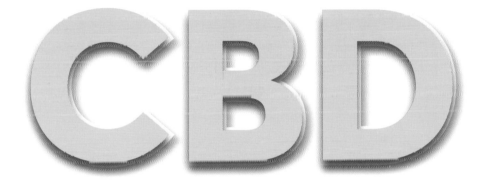

CENTENNIAL BOOKS

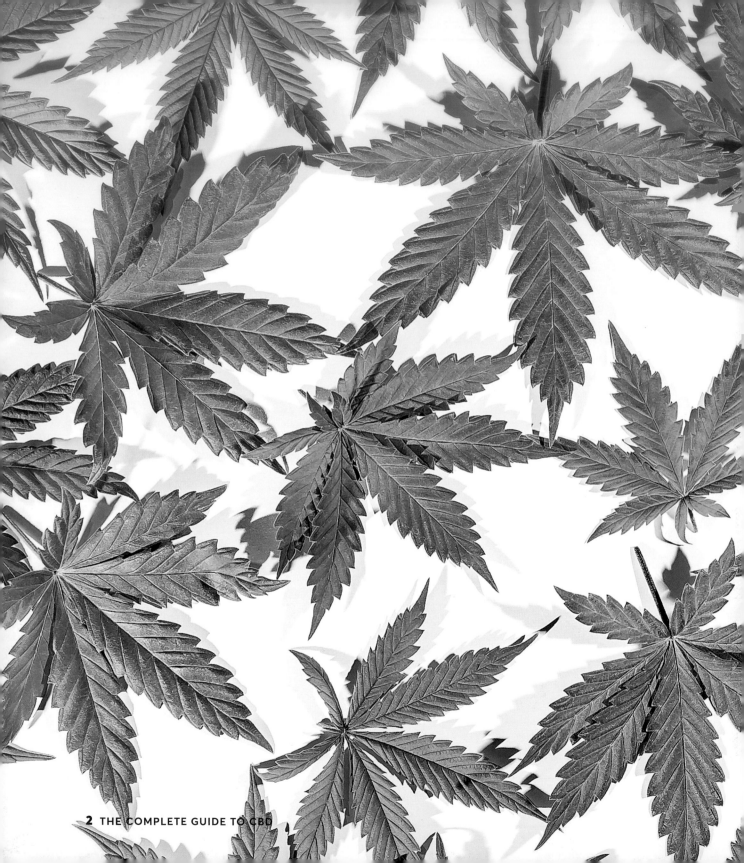

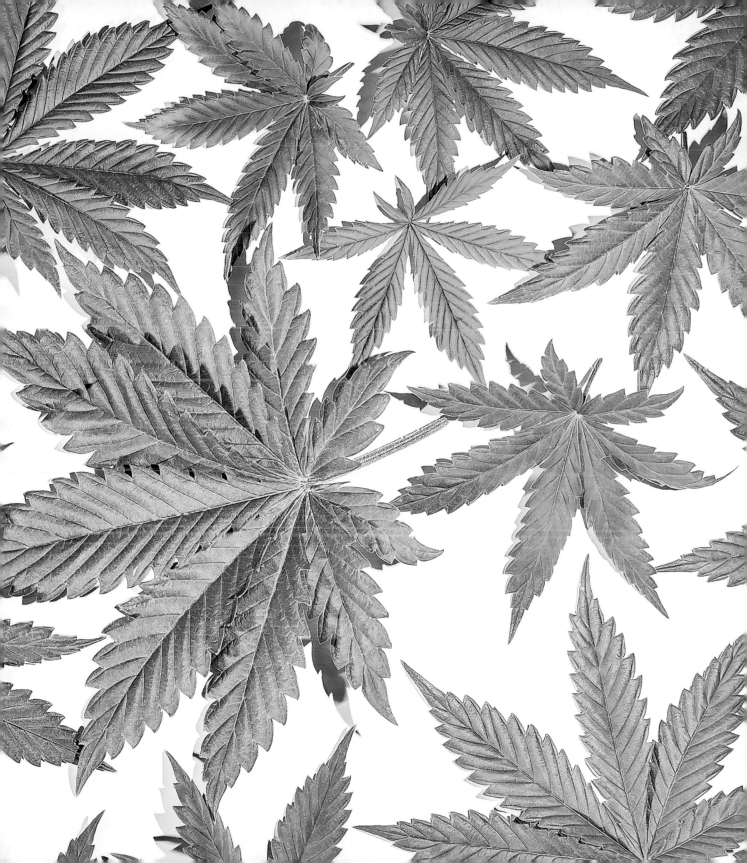

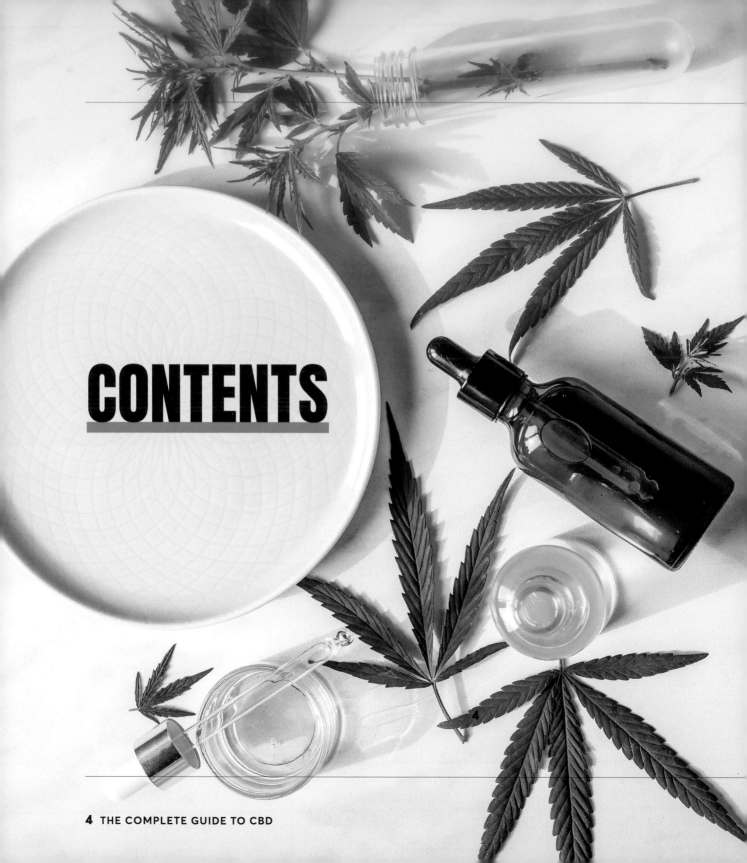

CONTENTS

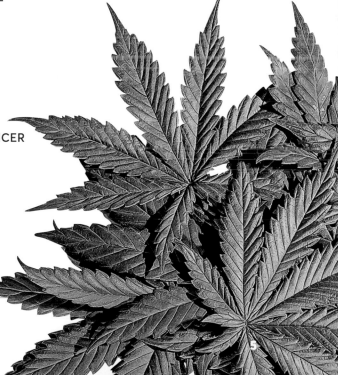

1

GETTING STARTED

CBD SEEMS TO BE THE TALK OF EVERY TOWN THESE DAYS. BUT BEFORE GIVING IT A TRY, IT'S A GOOD IDEA TO LEARN AS MUCH AS YOU CAN ABOUT THIS "MEDICAL MIRACLE," FROM WHAT IT IS TO HOW IT WORKS TO THE BEST WAYS TO CONSUME IT.

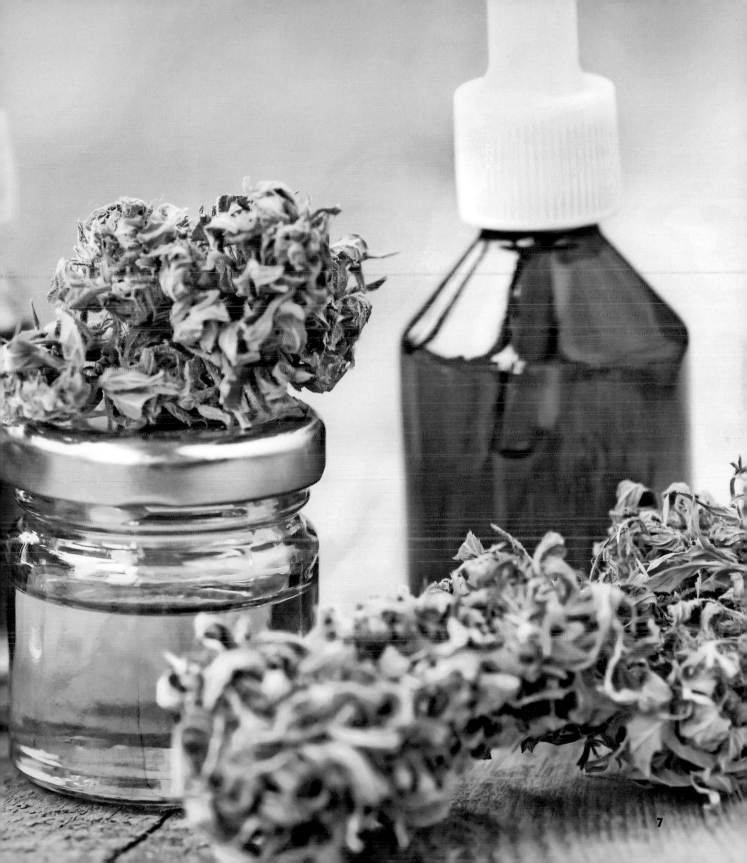

THE CBD EXPLOSION

What is it, really? And why is everyone going crazy over it now? Here is the complete story of CBD.

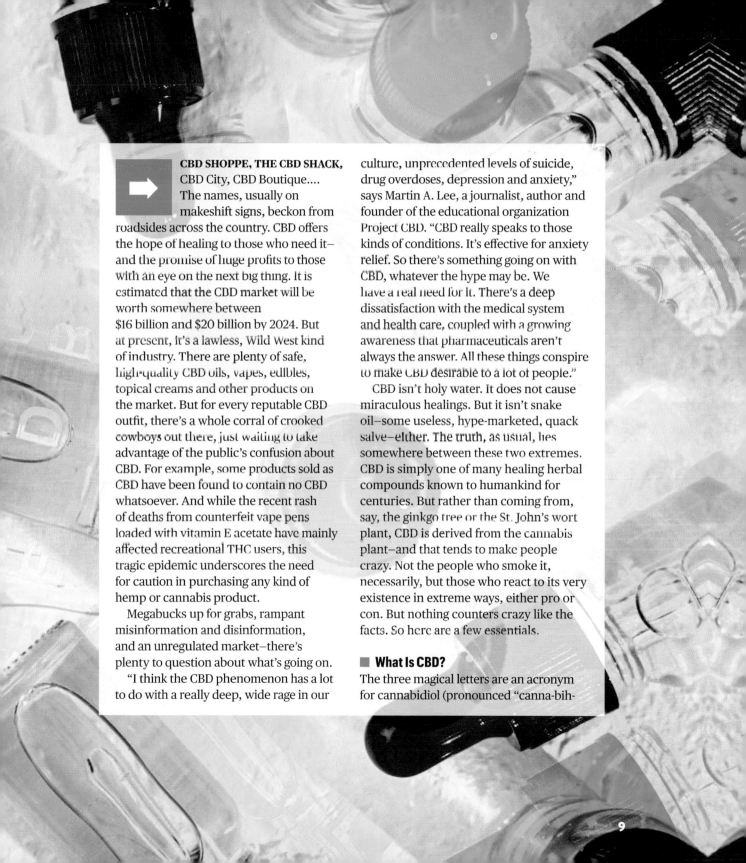

CBD SHOPPE, THE CBD SHACK, CBD City, CBD Boutique.... The names, usually on makeshift signs, beckon from roadsides across the country. CBD offers the hope of healing to those who need it—and the promise of huge profits to those with an eye on the next big thing. It is estimated that the CBD market will be worth somewhere between $16 billion and $20 billion by 2024. But at present, it's a lawless, Wild West kind of industry. There are plenty of safe, high-quality CBD oils, vapes, edibles, topical creams and other products on the market. But for every reputable CBD outfit, there's a whole corral of crooked cowboys out there, just waiting to take advantage of the public's confusion about CBD. For example, some products sold as CBD have been found to contain no CBD whatsoever. And while the recent rash of deaths from counterfeit vape pens loaded with vitamin E acetate have mainly affected recreational THC users, this tragic epidemic underscores the need for caution in purchasing any kind of hemp or cannabis product.

Megabucks up for grabs, rampant misinformation and disinformation, and an unregulated market—there's plenty to question about what's going on.

"I think the CBD phenomenon has a lot to do with a really deep, wide rage in our culture, unprecedented levels of suicide, drug overdoses, depression and anxiety," says Martin A. Lee, a journalist, author and founder of the educational organization Project CBD. "CBD really speaks to those kinds of conditions. It's effective for anxiety relief. So there's something going on with CBD, whatever the hype may be. We have a real need for it. There's a deep dissatisfaction with the medical system and health care, coupled with a growing awareness that pharmaceuticals aren't always the answer. All these things conspire to make CBD desirable to a lot of people."

CBD isn't holy water. It does not cause miraculous healings. But it isn't snake oil—some useless, hype-marketed, quack salve—either. The truth, as usual, lies somewhere between these two extremes. CBD is simply one of many healing herbal compounds known to humankind for centuries. But rather than coming from, say, the ginkgo tree or the St. John's wort plant, CBD is derived from the cannabis plant—and that tends to make people crazy. Not the people who smoke it, necessarily, but those who react to its very existence in extreme ways, either pro or con. But nothing counters crazy like the facts. So here are a few essentials.

What Is CBD?
The three magical letters are an acronym for cannabidiol (pronounced "canna-bih-

dye-all"), one of 483 chemical constituents of the cannabis plant, some 80 of which are classed as cannabinoids. Up until recently, CBD took a backseat to her more glamorous cannabinoid sister, THC (tetrahydrocannabinol). Rocketed to fame by the "reefer madness" paranoia of the 1930s, and beloved by the 1960s counterculture, THC is the stuff in pot that gets you high. CBD doesn't.

But the destigmatization and wider acceptance of cannabis over the past decade has helped shift the limelight onto the healing properties of CBD. Circa 2009, cultivators in Northern California—where cannabis has been medically legal since 1996 and fully legal since 2016—began breeding cannabis strains that were high in CBD rather than THC. A breeder named Lawrence Ringo was one of the pioneers in the field. And in 2011, the six Stanley brothers of Colorado developed what is probably the most well-known CBD strain, Charlotte's Web, named for Charlotte Figi, a childhood epilepsy sufferer who benefited greatly from CBD and has since become a poster child not only for CBD but for cannabis legalization in general.

■ Why Is CBD Suddenly So Hot?
The wheels of the current wave of CBD-mania were set in motion by the passage of the 2018 Agriculture Improvement Act, aka the Farm Bill. This legislation made it legal for farmers to grow hemp, which is simply cannabis that contains less than 0.3 percent of THC. Think of it as roughly analogous to the

difference between beer and "near beer." The latter is simply beer that has less than 0.5 percent alcohol by volume. Same stuff, but with a slightly different chemical makeup. Hence a different name—and one that seems less scary to certain segments of the population.

So, it became legal to sell products derived from hemp at a time when CBD was starting to impact the mainstream zeitgeist via stories like Charlotte Figi's. And from that parentage came a virtual license to print money.

According to a recent Consumer Reports study, some 64 million Americans have already taken CBD. Business leaders in the emergent and booming CBD space have tended to be companies entrenched in the recreational cannabis business in fully legal states like California, Colorado and Oregon. They are tooled up to switch some of their recreational grow over to a hemp-based CBD grow. And they've got the liquidity to expand into new acreage, not to mention fully geared-up product development and marketing teams. The beauty of CBD for these companies is that they're no longer

50%
Percentage of respondents in a Harris Poll of 2,000 CBD users who said they used it to reduce stress/anxiety.

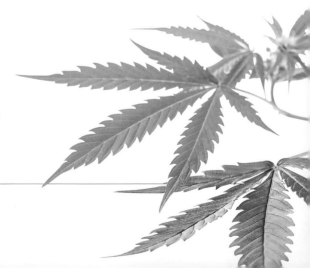

confined to selling only within state lines. Once they enter the hemp-based CBD market they can go nationwide, and with fewer of the costly legal and bureaucratic hassles that go with dealing in "marijuana."

One of the leaders in the CBD market is CannaCraft, a California company that has established a firm foothold in the THC recreational market. But CannaCraft CEO and founder Dennis Hunter says he has seen his CBD-only Care By Design product line grow exponentially in the past year. "It's about 35 percent of our business right now," he says. "By this time next year, it might be the majority of our grow. CBD has really caught on. It's really helpful and doesn't give people the psychoactive effect. People are finding relief from different products with CBD in them."

◼ CBD From Hemp vs. Marijuana

In some states you'll only legally be able to buy hemp-based CBD, which is definitely beneficial. But CBD can also be derived

from cannabis plants with more than 0.3 percent THC. This is known as whole-plant CBD, and it's generally held to be more beneficial than its hemp-based counterpart. This is due to a biochemical phenomenon known as the "entourage effect." CBD, THC and other cannabinoids interact in complex ways inside the body.

"CBD can be very effective, but sometimes it requires THC," says Sherry Yafai, MD, a Santa Monica, California-based physician who specializes in cannabis medicine. "THC opens up different doors in different receptors in the body than CBD does. And for pain, it can be very beneficial to open up these doors."

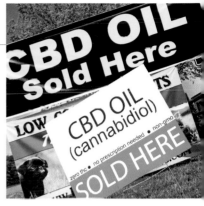

No matter where it comes from, CBD is CBD. On a molecular level, CBD from hemp is the same as CBD from marijuana.

While the FDA has not formally made statements for CBD's safety, the World Health Organization has provided data and stated that pure CBD is safe for consumption.

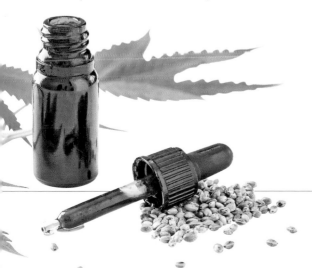

Good for What Ails You

A few conditions that CBD might help:

◼ EPILEPSY

This is where some of the most dramatic examples of CBD's efficacy have been seen. It has been particularly effective in treating two debilitating forms of epilepsy: Dravet syndrome and Lennox-Gastaut syndrome.

◼ PAIN

The anti-inflammatory and neuroprotective properties of CBD can help relieve pain, but it has generally been found to be more effective when taken in combination with THC. Inhaled and oral forms of CBD can decrease pain, but topical creams may also bring relief, as CBD penetrates the skin barrier better than THC.

◼ INSOMNIA

By helping decrease pain and anxiety, CBD can help you sleep better at night. It can also help regulate your circadian rhythms—the wake/sleep cycle.

■ ANXIETY/DEPRESSION

CBD can modify the permeability of some of our cells, which enables them to slow down the disintegration of certain chemicals in the body. These include the "feel good" neurotransmitters serotonin and anandamide (the "bliss molecule"). By slowing their breakdown, these neurochemicals stay in the body longer, helping to combat depression.

■ ADDICTION

Because of its effect on cell permeability, CBD can intensify the effects of certain opiates, so dosages can be reduced, diminishing the danger of overdose. There is also some indication that CBD can help people addicted to alcohol, nicotine and other substances better manage their cravings.

■ ALZHEIMER'S/PARKINSON'S/DEMENTIA

A few studies have indicated that CBD's neuroprotective properties may help with neurodegenerative diseases like Alzheimer's, Parkinson's or dementia.

In 2017, Yafai launched the ReLeaf Institute, where she treats patients and helms programs to educate physicians and the general public about medicinal cannabis. Also an adjunct instructor at the John Wayne Cancer Institute in LA, she put together a cancer support group, providing patients with information on the effectiveness of cannabis in relieving chemotherapy-related nausea, vomiting, anorexia and other debilitating side effects.

But one of the most dramatic examples she says she's seen of the combined healing power of CBD and THC was in a patient from South Carolina—we'll call him Patrick—who was severely addicted to prescription opioids. He'd traveled to California to consult with Yafai because medical cannabis was unavailable in his home state, and there were no qualified physicians with clinical cannabis experience. "He'd been on narcotics for over a decade," Yafai notes, "starting with a prescription from his doctor's office for low back pain. He was on about 50 to 80 milligrams of Percocet as well as oxytocin, and he was still having pain."

Like most people addicted to opioids, Patrick was constipated and sleep-deprived. "He was waking up at 2 or 4 in the morning just to take painkillers because he was having mini-withdrawals," Yafai relates. He had also entered a state of paranoia, another common side effect of opioid addiction. "He was carrying his three-month prescription of narcotics around on his back every day because he was afraid somebody was going to break into his house and steal them—that he would then be left with no prescription and the doctor wouldn't believe that he lost it or that somebody stole his prescription. So that fear and anxiety was almost married to his prescriptions—going to the pharmacist to pick up his prescription, having the pharmacist give him dirty looks every time.... His life started revolving around prescription painkillers—which, ultimately, weren't fixing the pain."

Yafai continues, "I got him off all the opioids in three months with a combination CBD/THC oil. Then he went off cannabis products and back to South Carolina feeling much better than he had in years—less pain, regular bowel movements and sleeping better."

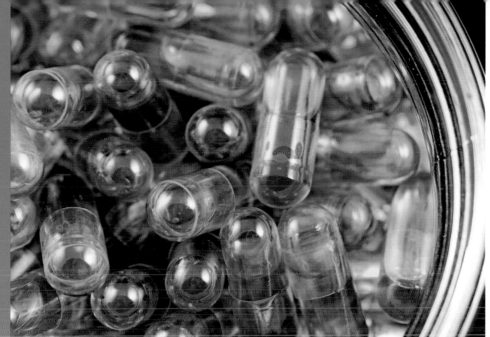

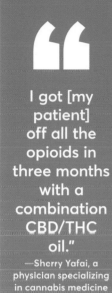

■ Dial In Your Dosage

When CBD alone doesn't seem to be working, a little THC can make a dramatic difference. Fortunately, there are many oil-based CBD products on the market that come in a variety of "strengths"–that is, a range of CBD to THC ratios. An oil with a 1:1 ratio will contain 50 percent CBD and 50 percent THC. Sativex–legal in Canada and parts of Europe–has a 1:1 ratio, which will produce a mild psychoactive effect. But lower ratios, like 18:1, won't. Other common ratios include 8:1, 4:1 and 3:1.

People's reactions vary, but the psychoactivity usually kicks in somewhere around 3:1–which can have its own therapeutic advantages in areas like pain relief. After all, medication like Xanax and a glass of wine both produce what's considered a "psychoactive effect"–and experts say cannabis is far less addictive than alprazolam or alcohol. Dosage ratios are also often key to treating serious

conditions like epilepsy. CannaCraft's Dennis Hunter recalled a patient who had suffered one or two seizures every day. A 4:1 ratio Care By Design oil helped her become seizure-free for a period of two months. "We went back and forth between the 8:1 and 4:1 and decided on the 4," he says. "The entourage effect really made a difference."

"Start low and go slow" is the universal rule in cannabis dosing. But that mainly applies to THC. The psychoactive effect can get a bit dark and disturbing at too high a dose. On the other hand, you can't really overdose on CBD, although you can definitely take more than you need. Rather, you're basically throwing your money away, like peeing out vitamins that your body hasn't been able to absorb.

Fortunately, those who work with CBD seem to agree on some rough dosage guidelines. "For an adult-sized person on no other medications, a low

39%

Percentage of 2,000 CBD users in a Harris Poll who said they used it to relieve chronic pain.

BACTERIAL INFECTION

A recent study by the University of Queensland in Australia has indicated that CBD may be helpful in combating the type of bacteria that causes dangerous diseases such as methicillin-resistant Staphylococcus aureus (MRSA), Streptococcus pneumoniae and E. faecalis. Many of these have become resistant to conventional antibiotics, which has tended to put people who are hospitalized at risk for contracting one of these diseases.

CANCER

No, CBD cannot cure cancer. But it can help relieve the side effects of chemotherapy, including nausea, vomiting, pain and anxiety.

ECZEMA/SKIN CONDITIONS

CBD administered orally and via topical creams can help relieve the itching, pain, swelling and other symptoms of skin diseases like eczema.

CAUTION!

Because CBD can affect the way certain drugs work in the body, it is strongly advised that you consult a physician before using CBD if you are currently on any other medications.

dose would be something like 5 to 10 milligrams," says Yafai.

"Over 30 or 40 milligrams, there's a point where you're not getting any effect," adds Hunter. "We've looked at research from Israel that confirms that. If somebody takes 200 milligrams of CBD, there may not be any benefit to it beyond 30 or 40 milligrams."

Which is an amazing thing about CBD—sometimes less of it is more powerful. "That cuts completely across the grain of how people think about medicine," says Martin Lee. "If it's a painkiller, you take more and it's better. With cannabis you don't have that. That's the kind of thing you have to keep in mind."

■ How Is CBD Consumed?

You can take CBD the same way you would all cannabis. The dried flower can be smoked, or a concentrate can be extracted from the plant matter, generally using CO_2, ethanol or some similar substance. This yields an oil that can be used in vape pens or made into a liquid taken sublingually. CBD can also be infused into tinctures, oils and butters without the use of chemicals. These infusions can be used to make edibles and topical creams for the skin.

"I generally use oils, tinctures and edibles more than anything else," says Yafai. "We use the inhalation route no more than probably 5 to 10 percent of the time. The reason is most of my patients are very sick and often at the extremes of age—very old or very young. I also use more oils because I can dose them better. I know what the patient is getting and we can dose two or three times a day—as opposed to smokable, where you have to inhale every two hours to get the effect, because the dosage wears off at around two hours. For people who have either mild anxiety or social situational anxiety, smoking is a great option. But for others, like a patient I have with cerebral palsy, autism and developmental delay, smoking is probably the worst option I could give him."

Our bodies are all different. There is no "one size fits all" dosage for any medicine. If you have a serious health condition, it's best to consult with a doctor or naturopath before using CBD. Unfortunately, trained physicians with extensive clinical cannabis experience are not always to be found. At present, cannabis isn't on the curriculum at many medical schools. Physicians like Yafai and Perry Solomon, medical adviser to the HelloMD website, have joined forces with organizations like the Society of Cannabis Clinicians to educate medical practitioners about cannabis. When you go to your family doctor with questions about CBD, you should be able to receive well-informed answers.

Naturopaths can also guide you toward a treatment plan. But for now, those of us in less cannabis-friendly states also have to be more self-reliant. One thing to look for in purchasing any CBD product is whether the CBD contained therein is a CBD isolate or a broad-spectrum or whole-plant CBD. This applies to both cannabis-based and hemp-based products. In an isolate, chemical extraction of the CBD is followed by an extensive process of filtering, refinement and pummeling whereby virtually all plant matter other than CBD is removed. This yields a fine white powder that is 99 percent pure CBD.

Lost in the isolate process, however, are healing, nonpsychoactive cannabinoids like CBN, CBC and CBG, as well as terpenes—aromatic plant secretions also known to have healing effects. This is one reason why many find broad-spectrum, whole-plant CBD products to be more effective. Of course, if you're in an area where only hemp-derived CBD is available, it's worth trying. Experts say it may still help your specific condition, and there's little downside beyond the expense.

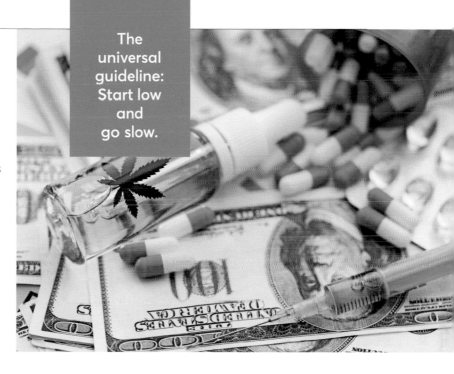

The universal guideline: Start low and go slow.

■ Can You Get Ripped Off?

Of course, as in any unregulated market, there's a possibility of fraud, and you may not be getting what you are paying for.

"Recently, I stumbled upon a product line, read the label and thought, 'Wow, this is really amazing; they are claiming 5000 milligrams of hemp CBD in a 10 milliliter bottle," says Yafai. "Lo and behold, when it was tested, it was actually 50 milligrams. So, there's a lot of discussion of how hemp CBD is trash, and the reason is because manufacturers poison the well...by not having good testing and good standards. And this is where I think the hemp market needs to start self-regulating to give itself that standard, because, unfortunately, the federal laws are always 10 steps behind."

According to statista.com, CBD consumer sales in the U.S. were estimated to be $813.2 million in 2019, up from $512.7 million in 2018.

"With this frenzy that's happening with CBD, a lot of companies are just jumping on the bandwagon and throwing some generic CBD from China into a product, just so they can list CBD on the label," Hunter adds. "Others don't even have CBD in them. We started testing products and a lot of them didn't have CBD in them."

So, in a way, purchasing CBD products is much like buying any herbal or homeopathic remedy. You have to do a bit of comparison shopping and networking with other customers to find the most reputable brands and the products that work best for you. Learn to look for spurious claims on labels. Also pay attention to what's not listed, as well as what is. The product itself can also give you a few clues.

"The more CBD or THC you have in an oil product, it increases the viscosity," says Yafai. "Meaning that the medication itself tends to be really thick. I've noticed that the stronger the medication is, the thicker the oil tends to be. If it's diluted, it tends to be a bit thinner. If you're taking oil that's fairly thin and it is advertising a very high dose, I would second-guess it."

Fortunately, there are companies like Confident Cannabis that will run lab tests on products for consumers. It isn't cheap, but it could be worth the expense in some cases. "If you or a loved one is going to be taking something for six months or more, I would consider getting it tested in a lab and see exactly what's in it, especially for a patient under 18," says Yafai. "Depending on

the legalities of the state where you live, you might have to send it out—which can be expensive, unfortunately."

■ Shouldn't Somebody Do Something About This?

CBD and medical cannabis fall under the jurisdiction of the U.S. Food and Drug Administration (FDA). As of the time of this writing, the GW Pharmaceuticals isolate Epidiolex is the only CBD product on the market that is approved by the FDA. But that situation is likely to change. On May 31, 2019, the FDA held a hearing on its Maryland campus titled "Scientific Data and Information About Products Containing Cannabis or Cannabis-Derived Compounds." One hundred twenty speakers, selected from an applicant pool of about 400, were each given either two or five minutes to make a presentation to a panel of FDA officials. This has been followed by further investigation, and the FDA has sent warning letters to several manufacturers of CBD products, advising them to stop making unfounded health claims in their labeling and marketing materials. The rash of recent vaping-related deaths and subsequent investigations will most likely motivate the FDA to act even more rapidly and decisively on this matter.

But the organization needs to base its actions on scientific data—something we don't have an abundance of right now, when it comes to CBD and cannabis-based medicine. Significant research has been done in countries like Israel and Canada. But it's hindered in the U.S. by the fact that

20%

Percentage of 2,000 CBD users in a Harris Poll who said they used it for migraine relief.

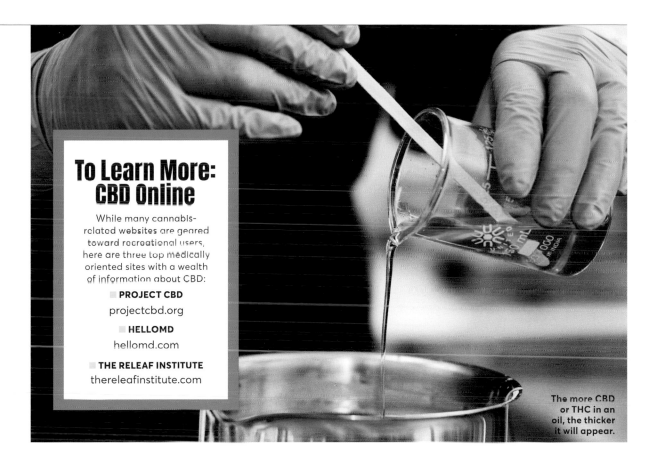

The more CBD or THC in an oil, the thicker it will appear.

cannabis is still classified as a Schedule 1 drug–"dangerous and with no perceived health benefit." And even where sufficient scientific data is available, the FDA approval process moves at a glacial pace. It is also not impervious to influence by lobbyists and other "interested parties." Many safe and valuable drugs become available in Europe a few years before receiving FDA approval. Meanwhile, dangerous opioids like Fentanyl get the fast track–the corporate VIP concierge lane.

So all eyes are on the 2020 election. If you'd like to see safe and reliable CBD products become more widely available, consider voting for politicians who advocate descheduling cannabis. Meanwhile, CBD will continue to offer healing to those who can shop wisely in a souk-like, swap meet kind of environment.

"Nobody can put the genie back in the bottle now," says Martin Lee. "There's no way they can cope with CBD by banning it or keeping it down."

THE KEYS TO CANNABIS

Marijuana and hemp may come from the same plant species, but they are very different in what they offer and how they are used. Grow your knowledge of how they vary here.

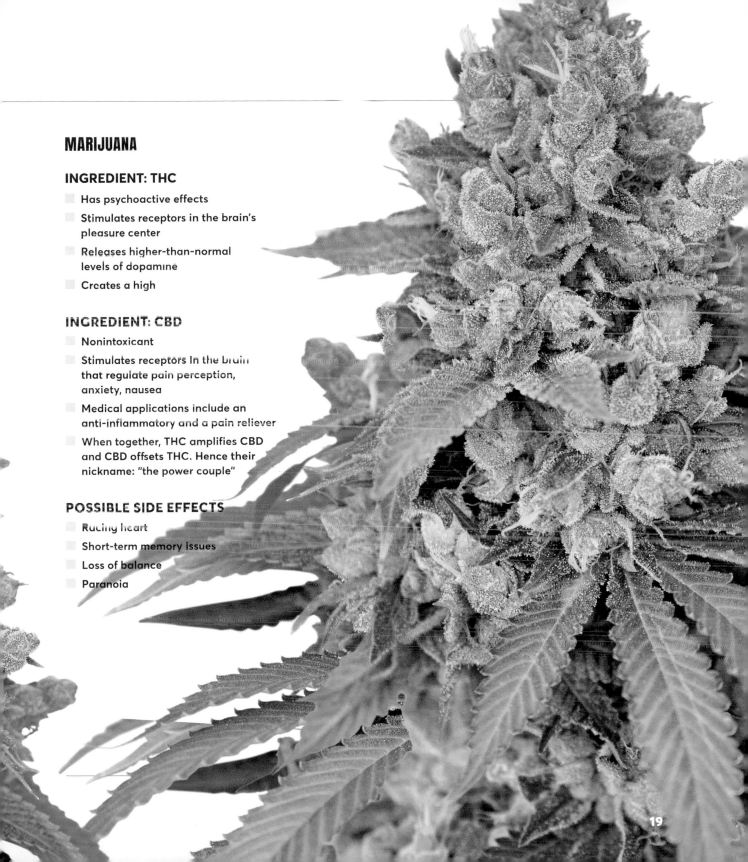

MARIJUANA

INGREDIENT: THC

- Has psychoactive effects
- Stimulates receptors in the brain's pleasure center
- Releases higher-than-normal levels of dopamine
- Creates a high

INGREDIENT: CBD

- Nonintoxicant
- Stimulates receptors in the brain that regulate pain perception, anxiety, nausea
- Medical applications include an anti-inflammatory and a pain reliever
- When together, THC amplifies CBD and CBD offsets THC. Hence their nickname: "the power couple"

POSSIBLE SIDE EFFECTS

- Racing heart
- Short-term memory issues
- Loss of balance
- Paranoia

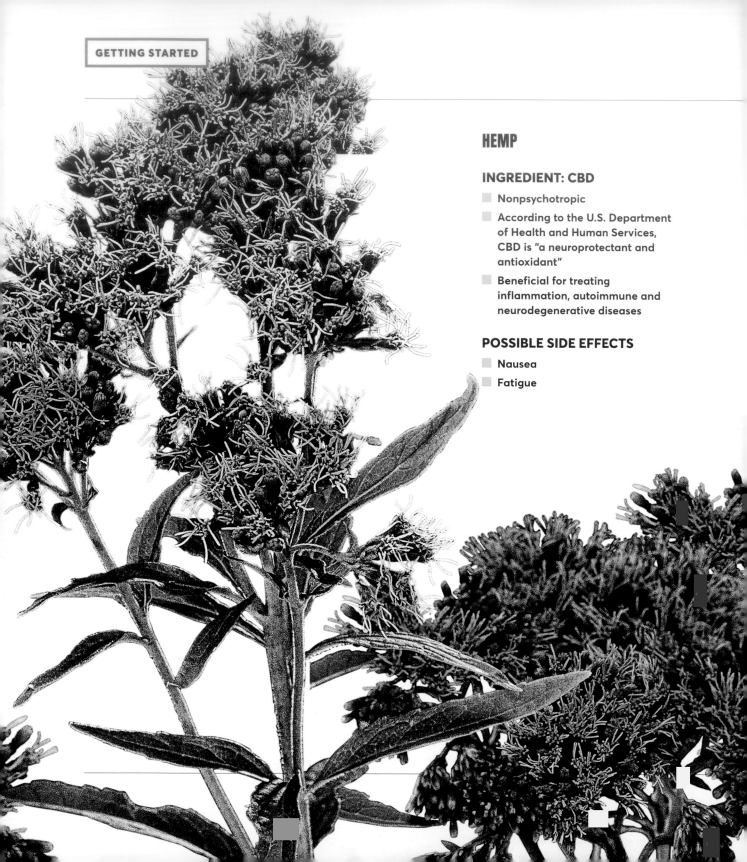

HEMP

INGREDIENT: CBD

- Nonpsychotropic
- According to the U.S. Department of Health and Human Services, CBD is "a neuroprotectant and antioxidant"
- Beneficial for treating inflammation, autoimmune and neurodegenerative diseases

POSSIBLE SIDE EFFECTS

- Nausea
- Fatigue

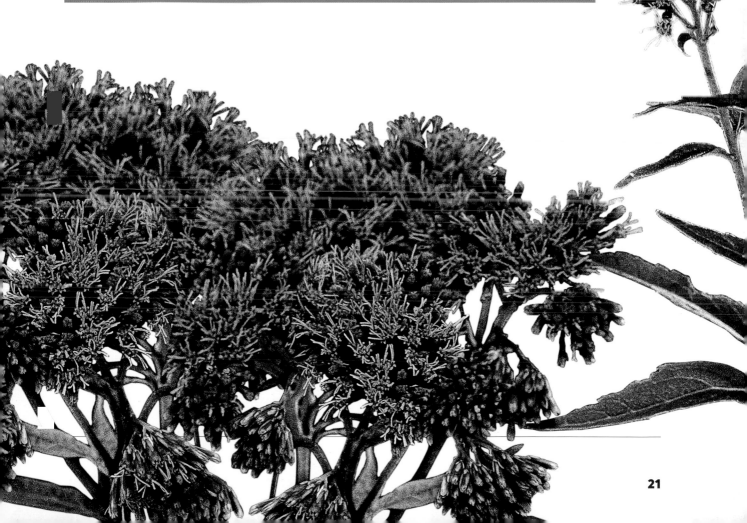

CBD Label Facts

Get to know the differences between hemp oil, CBD oil, hemp extract and CBD extract, as well as full-spectrum and CBD isolate.

1 / HEMP OIL
Cold pressed from the seed

2 / CBD OIL
Extracted from the flowers. Some companies label CBD oil (extract) as hemp oil in order to navigate regulation. Look for the words CBD, extract or hemp extract on a label. The product should contain CBD, because the "extract" is from hemp flowers (where cannabinoids are produced).

3 / FULL-SPECTRUM CBD
Contains CBD and other minor cannabinoids (may include THC).

4 / CBD ISOLATE
Contains 99.9 percent CBD and no other cannabinoids.

TO CBD OR NOT TO CBD?

The scientific studies are still skimpy, but here's what we do know about this potentially miraculous medicine.

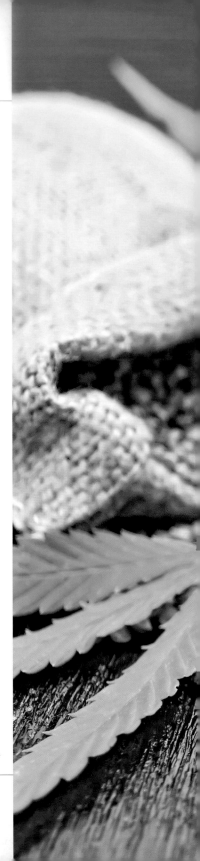

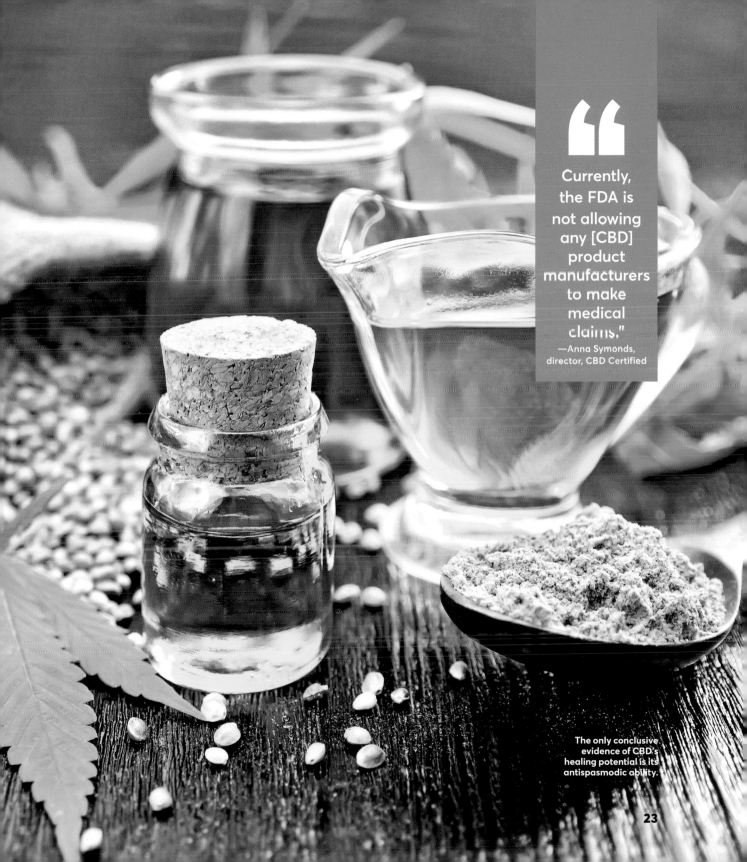

> " Currently, the FDA is not allowing any [CBD] product manufacturers to make medical claims."
> —Anna Symonds, director, CBD Certified

The only conclusive evidence of CBD's healing potential is its antispasmodic ability.

THINK OF CBD PRODUCTS as the Kardashians of the health and wellness world: It seems like everyone talks about them all the time, but at the end of the day, most of us still don't know much about exactly what it is they do.

This is all happening despite the fact that the plant that delivers most of our CBD–cannabis–is still illegal under federal guidelines, which means conclusive medical research on its effects is hard to come by. For the moment, therefore, CBD mania is based largely on word of mouth about what the medicine can do. That seems very familiar for Shira Adler: The author of *The ABCs of CBD: The Essential Guide for Parents (And Regular Folks Too)* and founder of the health and wellness company Synergy by Shira Adler recalls a time not so long ago when another natural cure was the Next Big Thing.

"Remember 10 or 15 years ago, when echinacea wasn't a thing but became a thing?" she says. "I think of CBD like that. Back in the day, nobody knew what echinacea was unless they'd been exposed to some sort of homeopathic or naturopathic treatment. I don't know what broke it but it became a main way to support the immune system. CBD has done the same thing, which is very significant and I'm glad it's becoming the biggest buzzworthy word in health and wellness in a decade because it paves the way for more awareness."

But what exactly should consumers be aware of? Here are answers to some common questions you might have about CBD, before you give it a try:

■ There's so much discussion of CBD now, but what exactly is it?

Technically, CBD stands for "cannabidiol," one of more than 100 identified molecules in hemp and cannabis plants, according to Anna Symonds, director of the Oregon-based educational organization CBD Certified. Although people have spent thousands of years using the entire cannabis plant for both its medicinal and mind-altering effects, it wasn't until the 1960s that Israeli scientist Dr. Raphael Mechoulam became the first to map and describe the structure of the CBD molecule.

■ The stories about CBD all seem pretty miraculous, but what are some issues that it can help me with?

First, it's important to remember that scientists have yet to prove very much when it comes to CBD's healing powers. Explains Symonds, "We need much more research and more clinical trials." However, veteran cannabis industry educator/consultant Emma Chasen notes that there has been conclusive evidence regarding CBD's antispasmodic and anti-epileptic abilities. In addition, preclinical studies have found CBD may also be an anti-inflammatory, an analgesic, a muscle relaxer, an antidepressant and an immunity modulator. Meanwhile, there's plenty

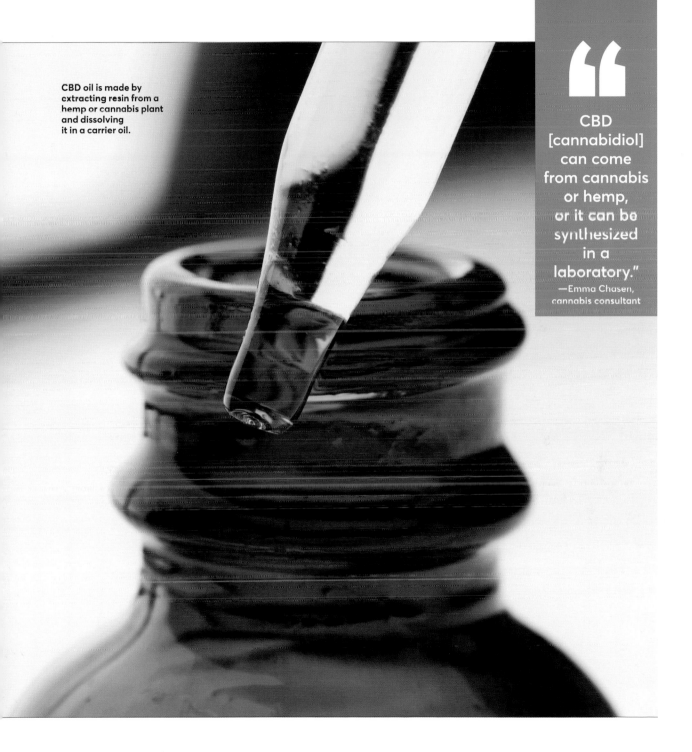

CBD oil is made by extracting resin from a hemp or cannabis plant and dissolving it in a carrier oil.

"
CBD [cannabidiol] can come from cannabis or hemp, or it can be synthesized in a laboratory."
—Emma Chasen, cannabis consultant

of anecdotal evidence that it has helped sufferers of everything from psoriasis to anorexia to insomnia to Parkinson's.

▪ It seems almost too good to be true. So how does it do what it does to our bodies once we take it?

Every part of us—from our brains to our internal organs to our respiratory and muscular systems—has what are called CBD receptors. These soak up the CBD, which Adler says "just knows what is out of whack. It addresses your deficiency points and what is causing them." CBD is "a very promiscuous compound," adds Chasen.

"It can interact with many different receptor families and factors in the body, initiating a variety of physiological responses, all with the goal of maintaining homeostasis [a state of equilibrium within the body]."

▪ Is there a difference between a hemp plant and a cannabis plant when it comes to buying CBD?

Not exactly, although they are related. "Hemp is a kissing cousin of the

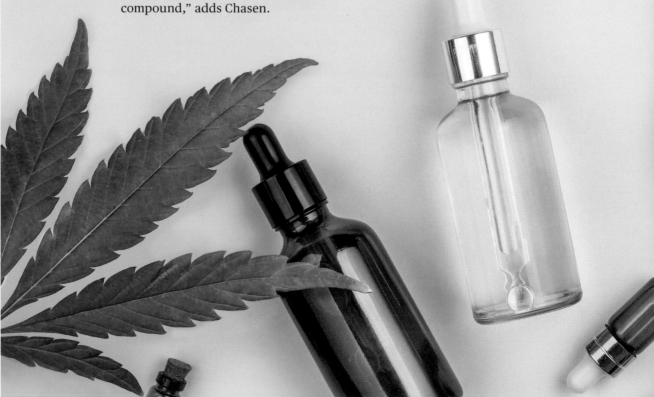

cannabis plant," says Adler. Morris Beegle, president of We Are For Better Alteratives (WAFBA) and founder of the NoCo Hemp Expo, the world's largest hemp conference and exhibition, admits telling the difference between the two can be confusing, since "hemp is one molecule compound away from the cannabis plant." For cannabis to be considered hemp, it legally has to have less than 0.3 percent of the intoxicating cannabinoid THC. This essentially means hemp-based CBD, which is legal across the country, is more like a vitamin than a medicine, while "the CBD in dispensaries in legal states comes from the cannabis side," Beegle explains.

■ **When using a medicine that's strictly CBD, will I be able to avoid getting "high"?**
Completely. It doesn't have the intoxication properties that THC does. However, people wrongly assume that CBD is "nonpsychoactive," says Symonds. "While it's nonintoxicating, it is in fact psychoactive–it interacts with our nervous system to produce changes in mood and/or behavior, including anti-anxiety and antipsychotic [symptoms]. So it won't get you high, but it's a good thing that it's psychoactive, because we can gain therapeutic effects through these pathways."

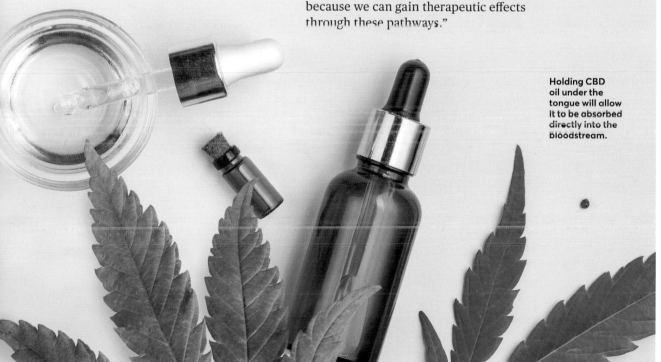

Holding CBD oil under the tongue will allow it to be absorbed directly into the bloodstream.

Seeding Is Believing

Hemp seed oil isn't CBD, but it can still be helpful. As the CBD phenomenon continues to flourish, it's hard enough for consumers to learn the difference between hemp-derived CBD oils and cannabis-derived CBD oils. To make it even more confusing, though, many companies have also stepped up the marketing of what they call "hemp seed oil." So what are the differences between all of these treatments? Cannabis educator/consultant Emma Chasen explains it this way: "Hemp-derived CBD products can be efficacious in managing a variety of symptoms. However, it's very important to examine the source of hemp and the product formulation practices. Cannabis-derived CBD may be the most efficacious in managing symptoms due to the rigorous analytical testing requirements. Hemp seed oil does not contain CBD, so it will not have much therapeutic potential."

Still, that doesn't mean it's without any healing powers. "Hemp seed oil is generally recognized as something safe to take, like echinacea or lavender," says Morris Beegle, president and co-founder of We Are For Better Alternatives (WAFBA).

"The seeds have a lot of nutritional value, like flax or chia seeds...very high in protein and omega 3, 6 and 9. Humans have been eating them for a long time, probably thousands of years, long before we knew what CBD was."

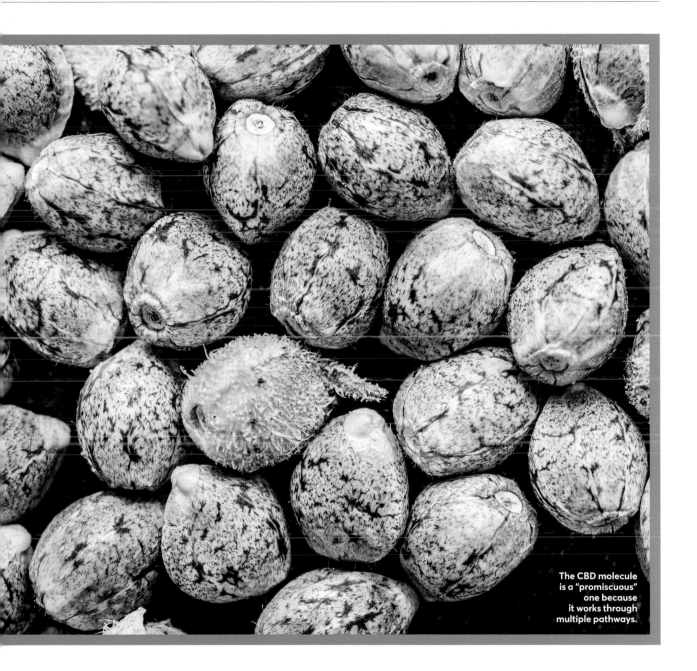

The CBD molecule is a "promiscuous" one because it works through multiple pathways.

AS YOU LIKE IT

When it comes to figuring out how to best consume or apply CBD, there are now many options to suit your needs.

There's no doubt we live in an era of seemingly unlimited choices. Whether you're looking for a TV show to watch, someone to deliver your Chinese food or a cellular company to keep you steeped in Wi-Fi, you can easily get overwhelmed with service options. CBD is no different. There was a time when cannabis was simply that funny-smelling stuff you smoked or your roommate's hippie friend baked into brownies. As interest in cannabidiol increases, though, so do the methods for consuming it. Here is a look at both the benefits and the drawbacks of the most popular ways to indulge.

23%

Percentage drop in the purchases of cannabis flower products in Colorado in the first four years

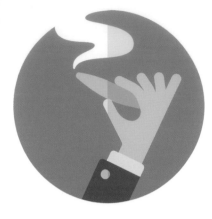

Smoking

Once the only game in town, it's still a popular way to get high —if that's your goal. However, if you're more interested in the healing effects of CBD than the intoxicating effects of THC, smoking is the wrong move. According to Jim Walsh, a veteran cannabis public relations specialist whose clients include industry leader Bloom Farms, very little marijuana flower in the U.S. has much CBD. Which means "there are much better ways to go at this stage if CBD is what you want," he explains.

Edibles

Whether it's in a gummy bear, a cookie or a chocolate bar, eating your CBD is fast becoming the most popular form of consumption. Still, it must pass through your liver before it can head off to do its thing, which can mean an onset time of between 20 minutes and two hours, explains Walsh. However, once it does get going, the CBD can work for up to four or five hours. "This can lead to a common error," Walsh says. "People take a little, think it's not working, then take more—which you shouldn't do."

Supplements

These "aren't that common right now, but they're getting there," explains Walsh. They are sort of a multivitamin for this cannabis era, providing a synergistic effect by combining CBD with other healthy ingredients. These "cocktails of things that are beneficial for people," he adds, will most likely have the same onset time as an edible, since they go through the same route in the body. However, "these are still very new, so it's hard to say. That's why it's important to buy them from a reputable brand you already trust."

Vaping

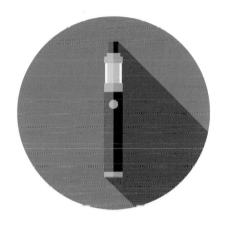

This can be done in two different ways: with a vape pen, or a larger vaporizer (like your mom used to put in your room when you had a bad cold). The primary benefit is the rapid onset of the effects, which can hit you in as few as five minutes. The downsides? There's a lot unknown about the safety of vaping, especially with the rash of illnesses and deaths associated with this method. Plus, Walsh says it can be hard to find a pen that effectively delivers CBD, and the effect usually fades within 90 minutes.

Topicals

Think lotions, creams, salves and bath bombs, all of which are gaining in popularity these days. The CBD in these treatments can start treating conditions in five to 15 minutes in many cases, because the topicals are usually being applied to the precise location where you need help. That's great news for people dealing with conditions involving inflammation, such as fibromyalgia and rheumatoid arthritis. However, adds Walsh, the skin will absorb some of the product, possibly limiting CBD's ability to fully treat patients.

Ingestibles

This includes tinctures—drops you put under your tongue—and sublinguals—things like mints that you hold in your mouth as they dissolve. Both can quickly move into your bloodstream. The onset time from a tincture dropper, according to Walsh, can be around 30 minutes, with the effects lasting about as long as an edible. Sublinguals, meanwhile, could possibly get to work within seven to 10 minutes. "[Ingestibles] offer some level of consistency in dosing," says Walsh. "That's what I personally like about them."

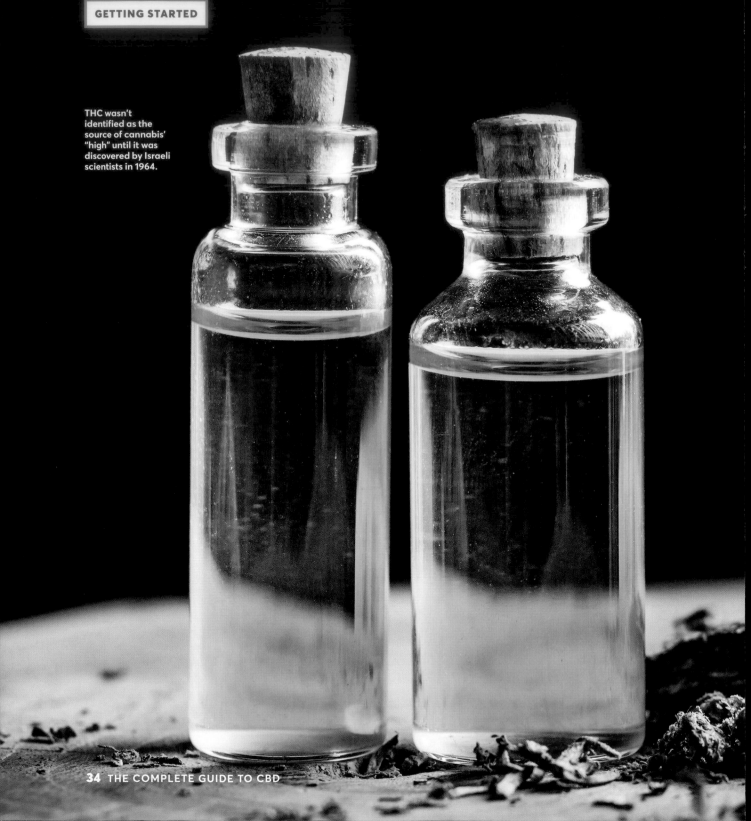

THC wasn't identified as the source of cannabis' "high" until it was discovered by Israeli scientists in 1964.

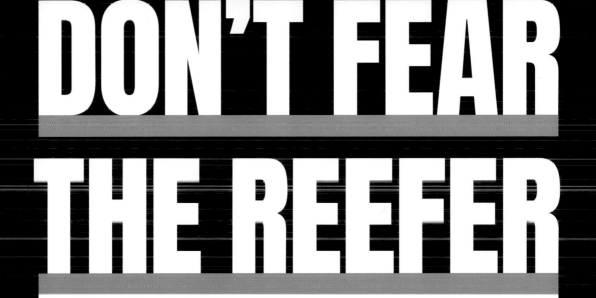

DON'T FEAR THE REEFER

Worries about the psychoactive THC may be keeping people from cannabis—but in appropriate doses it can have a positive impact.

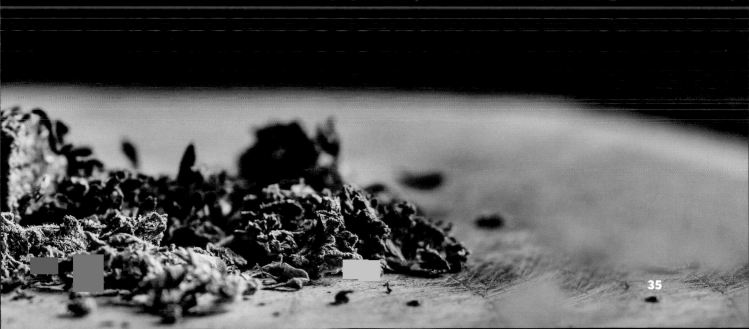

There is really no better revelation of how old we've become than the way we think about using marijuana.

In your late teens and 20s, if you're into cannabis, the whole point is to get high. The more THC in whatever you're smoking, the better. A few kids, mortgages and bouts of sciatica later, though, and chances are your interests have done a complete 180. Now, if you're considering cannabis at all, it's probably for the relaxing, healing powers of CBD. The thought of experiencing a good old-fashioned THC high can actually be downright terrifying.

It's perfectly understandable that adults with plenty of responsibilities, as well as plenty of memories of their behavior while stoned in college, might hesitate to indulge in THC even in states where it's now legal. After all, this psychoactive cannabinoid is not only what's responsible for the legendary high feeling that has made marijuana so popular over the years—according to cannabis industry educator and consultant Emma Chasen, it's also an ingredient that might produce plenty of unwanted issues.

"If overdosed, it can cause uncomfortable side effects such as anxiety, paranoia, elevated heart rate and impaired memory," she explains.

Still, living in fear of THC may well be a mistake. For starters, indulging in too much of it "can't physiologically kill you," Chasen says. "Plus, it has potential as an analgesic, specifically when targeting radicular pain [like sciatica] or pain tied to emotional trauma, such as PTSD."

Even more significant than THC's solo effects, though, is what the most abundant cannabinoid in the cannabis matrix can do when combined with the second-most abundant cannabinoid, CBD. When they work together, Chasen explains, they can possibly provide "extraordinary medical benefits" because they amplify each other's medicinal properties. This balance of both substances can help keep any uncomfortable THC side effects at bay.

■ A Dynamic Duo

"A lot of people choose products that contain CBD isolate rather than full-spectrum oil because the CBD isolate does not contain any THC," says Chasen. "The frustrating thing is that the full-spectrum oil will most likely work better than the CBD isolate without delivering any psychotropic experience—if the THC concentration is low enough compared to CBD."

"They work synergistically," adds Oleg MaryAces, director of education and marketing for Brooklyn, New York-based cannabis company Lock & Key Remedies. "In some ways, they improve each other's functionality. CBD affects THC in that it takes away some of the psychoactivity on a molecular level."

Take depression and anxiety, for instance, two maladies that MaryAces admits he's suffered from. He knew that THC had antidepressant properties but at the same time, it could potentially exacerbate anxiety. "Even if it cools you off, it can start shaking up your system," he says. "And I didn't want that feeling of getting high because it's detrimental to me being functional." At the same time, he knew that CBD reportedly eases symptoms of anxiety, but hasn't been as productive in elevating people coping with depression. So, putting them together provided what he calls "a nice balance."

According to Chasen, a THC and CBD combo has also been known to provide relief for ailments like digestive disorders, inflammation, immune disorders, neuropathic pain and chemotherapy side effects such as nausea and vomiting. Turning these two cannabinoids into a dynamic duo requires a fair amount of time and effort, however. It's critical to find the perfect amount of each for your own body so neither overpowers the other—or provides no relief at all.

"Education is the key to getting it right," says MaryAces. "If you're going to consume THC for the first time, you have to know your dose and make sure it's a small dose. You don't want to shock your system. And with CBD, you also have to start slow because you don't want to take more of something when you don't need it. Then increase the amount until you feel a benefit."

■ Boosting the Bud
"Because cannabis medicine is highly personalized, it takes experimentation to find the ratio to produce the experience you desire," Chasen adds. "If you're new

to cannabis and want to experiment with mixed ratios, start with 10mg CBD plus 2.5mg THC. Increase the CBD dose by 5mg increments and the THC dose by 2.5mg increments until you reach a dose that delivers the experience you want."

CBD isn't just giving THC a boost to help whatever ails you. It's also elevating its fellow cannabinoid's reputation.

"CBD has done a good job of demythologizing THC," explains MaryAces. "The benefits from using them together are making THC feel less taboo." Adds Chasen, "With the CBD movement's rise in popularity, people are coming to accept cannabis and hemp. We should use this cultural momentum to encourage an investigation of the benefits of including THC in the mix with CBD."

Cannabis Tip

"A THC and CBD combo has been known to provide relief for ailments like digestive disorders, inflammation, immune disorders, neuropathic pain and chemotherapy side effects such as nausea and vomiting."

—Emma Chasen, cannabis industry educator

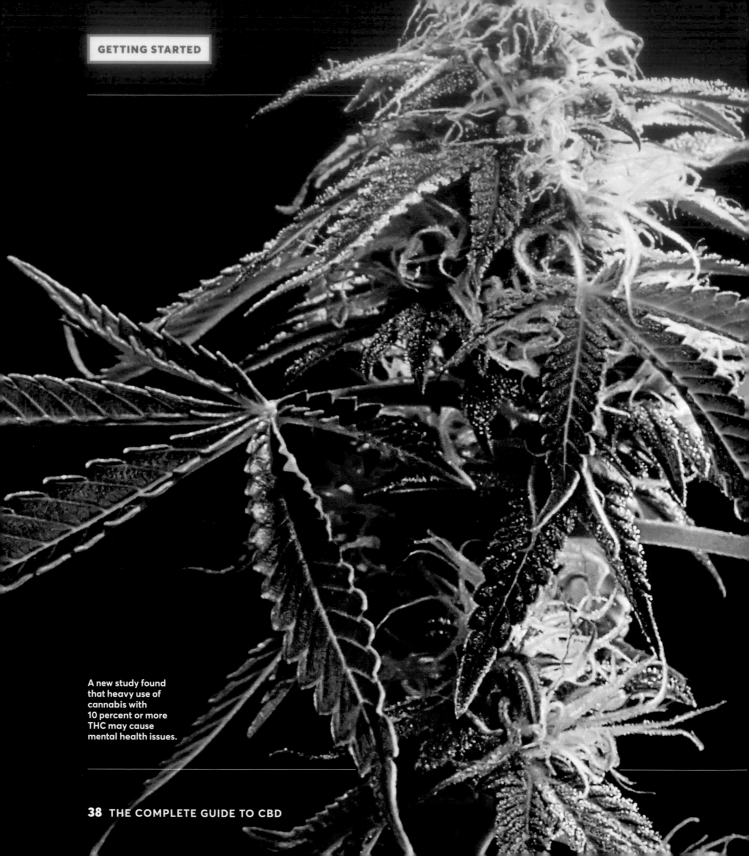

A new study found that heavy use of cannabis with 10 percent or more THC may cause mental health issues.

When THC Met CBD

How do these two cannabinoids interact to benefit our bodies in a way they can't on their own? We asked cannabis consultant and educator Emma Chasen to describe the process.

"THC and CBD amplify each other's medicinal properties, and the balance typically helps keep any uncomfortable side effects at bay. This may be explained by the way in which THC and CBD interact with our CB1 receptors. CB1 receptors are part of our endocannabinoid receptor systems. They exist primarily in the brain and can signal for different pathways when engaged. THC engages the CB1 receptor at the main binding site and signals for many pathways including anxiolytic (anti-anxiety), analgesic, anti-inflammatory and psychotropic activity. CBD does not effectively bind to the CB1 receptor on its own, but it can when THC is already bound to the main binding site.

"When THC engages the CB1 receptor at the main binding site, it opens up a secondary location on that same receptor that CBD can bind to. When both THC and CBD are bound to the same CB1 receptor, the medicinal signaling pathways are amplified and the psychotropic activity diminishes. In this way, CBD acts as a kind of EpiPen for the uncomfortable side effects of THC."

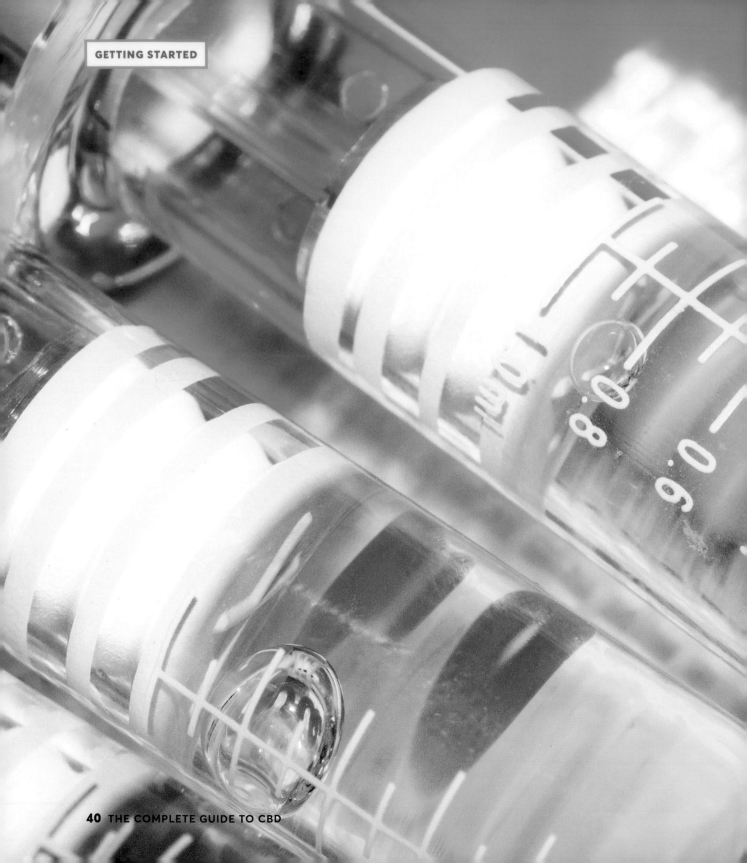

LESS IS MORE

If you're using cannabis for health, take into account just how much THC may be in whatever you're consuming.

GIVEN ALL THE ATTENTION it's getting these days, CBD is clearly A-OK for millions of Americans when it comes to battling a variety of ailments. However, its cannabis counterpart–THC–can be just as helpful when treating many illnesses. That's why many dispensaries offer medicines that provide an "entourage effect"–combining the benefits of both CBD and THC to improve their customer's health. There's just one thing for people to be aware of, though: The strength of today's THC is far beyond what consumers may remember from their college days.

Take Oregrown, for instance. The company's flagship dispensary in Bend, Oregon, offers 31 strains of cannabis with THC levels above 20 percent and just five that are below. While the majority of its customers are looking for flower with power, Oregrown's co-founder and chief brand officer, Chrissy Hadar, isn't one of them.

"I'm a business owner and a mother," she says. "I'm really busy. I want something that just kind of helps me chill out at night so I prefer something that's more in the teens with a little CBD. Not everybody wants a super-high-testing THC strain. There are plenty of customers out there looking for lower testing strains, but it falls heavily on the dispensary and customer service to educate clients on the positives."

■ The "Entourage Effect"

Just like there are wine snobs, experts suggest we need to become marijuana snobs–in a good way. There's so much more to the plant than just THC, which is just one of the hundreds of cannabinoids and terpenes that can help you get to your happy place. Unless all you care about is getting as stoned as possible, the key is to think about how you want to feel. Thanks to that aforementioned "entourage effect," it's possible to really fine-tune the high and medicinal benefits you want. All it takes is a certain sophistication.

"THC is just one 'must' metric out of hundreds of metrics," says Hadar. "It doesn't take into account all of the other cannabinoids present in the plant, and most specifically the terpene profile, which is really what is going to dictate the type of high you get from it" because of its sedative properties, for instance.

"Just because something tests really high in THC doesn't mean that it's going to give you the desired high you're looking for," she continues. "The best advice is to ask questions and look past the test results displayed next to the flower. If you have an idea of the kind of high you're looking for, I would stay away from looking at numbers and focus more on the cannabinoids, the terpenes, the look and smell of the flower."

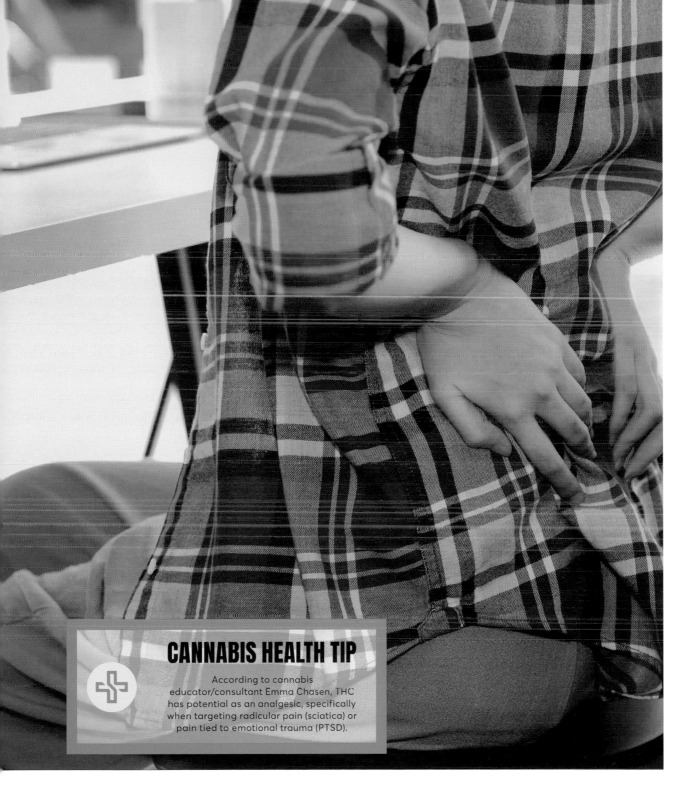

CANNABIS HEALTH TIP

According to cannabis educator/consultant Emma Chasen, THC has potential as an analgesic, specifically when targeting radicular pain (sciatica) or pain tied to emotional trauma (PTSD).

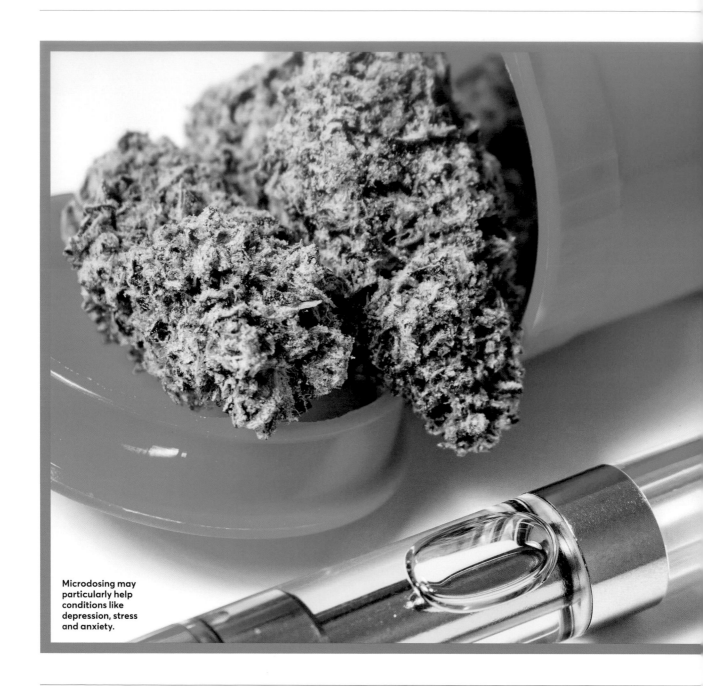

Microdosing may particularly help conditions like depression, stress and anxiety.

Small Doses, Big Results?

While the talk about THC and CBD these days is all about getting larger percentages of it into strains, that's also led to a growing philosophy promoting the use of smaller amounts of both: microdosing. Basically, this approach entails obtaining the medical benefits of THC, along with its cannabinoid cousins, while being able to function normally in your daily life. Smaller dosages at regular intervals can actually produce more of the desired effects than ingesting massive quantities at different times. Meanwhile, according to experts, any undesired psychoactive effects will be minimal or nonexistent. A little THC can help make you more mindful, less irritable and more focused—and who doesn't want that during their day?

Bear in mind, however, that what qualifies as "microdosing" for one person might not work the same magic for another. It all depends on your own tolerance and your chemical makeup. Experimentation is the key, but cannabis experts recommend taking a two-day hiatus from weed if you're a regular user and then starting with 2.5 milligrams of THC for three days before increasing it (if necessary) in order to see what the right microdose is for you. Although you could take a puff or two off a vape pen, the best way to do it is with tinctures, oils or edibles made specifically for it, since you can more easily control the dosage.

SERVING UP CBD

As for CBD microdosing, the starting doses can be higher, according to cannabis industry consultant and educator Emma Chasen. She has found that "consumers usually feel symptoms of relief at around 10mg to 20mg of CBD. Negative side effects associated with [CBD] are incredibly rare, so the likelihood of an uncomfortable experience is fairly low."

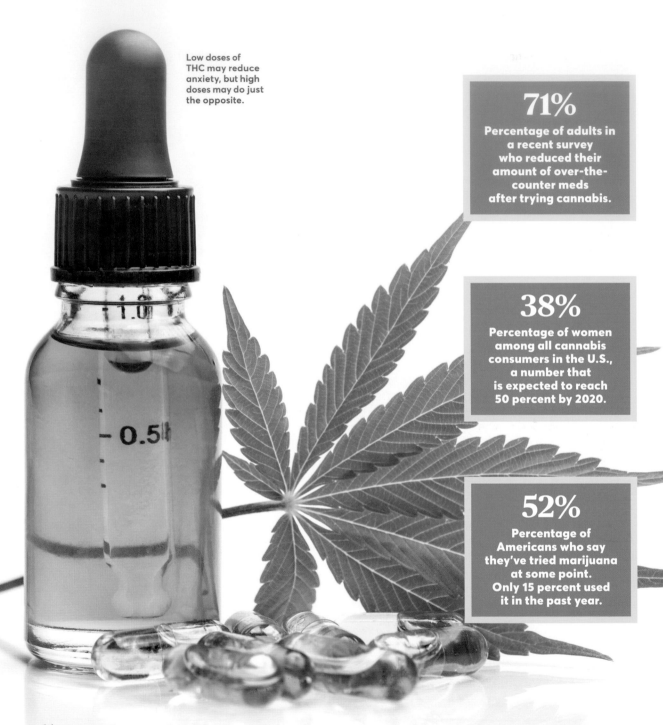

Low doses of THC may reduce anxiety, but high doses may do just the opposite.

71%
Percentage of adults in a recent survey who reduced their amount of over-the-counter meds after trying cannabis.

38%
Percentage of women among all cannabis consumers in the U.S., a number that is expected to reach 50 percent by 2020.

52%
Percentage of Americans who say they've tried marijuana at some point. Only 15 percent used it in the past year.

■ Creating Combinations

These days, of course, many customers are viewing cannabis as more than just a way to get high. They also want it to help with their overall wellness. That's why Oregrown's menu features plenty of strains that provide both the intoxicating feeling that comes with THC and the health benefits of CBD. Their list includes items like AC/DC Cookies, with 10 percent THC and 11 percent CBD; Pineapple Yeager, 8 percent THC and 14 percent CBD; and Sugar Plum, 11 percent THC and 4 percent CBD—all of which are produced by East Fork Cultivars in southern Oregon. These combinations can help with everything from pain relief to insomnia to inflammation to anxiety.

"We do really well with low-THC strains as long as they have a significant amount of CBD in them," says Hadar, noting that Oregrown doesn't even publish the THC percentage next to its flower display. "It's on our menu, but it's not something we are focused on since the day we opened our doors. We want the customers to smell the flower and ask questions about the terpene profile and total cannabinoids. We want to have the opportunity to educate them instead of them just being number-chasers looking for highest THC content."

While too much THC can be a bad thing, the opposite is generally not true when it comes to CBD. Higher levels of cannabidiol are not an issue, according to Oleg MaryAces, who runs a Brooklyn, New York, health and wellness company, Lock & Key Remedies, which specializes in high-potency hemp oils that feature a significant amount of CBD.

■ Spiking the CBD

"There's been a major push in the past four or five years of crossbreeding strains to lower the THC content and increase the CBD content as much as possible," says MaryAces, who is seeing strains with CBD in the 12 percent to 15 percent range, compared to 3 percent to 5 percent a decade ago. "As long as you're not taking any kind of blood thinner like Warfarin, for example, for the average person, there's no negative side effects with high CBD strains—whereas if you take too much THC, like in an edible, you could have one of the worst experiences of your life."

And that, in a nutshell, is what it all comes down to—recreating the desired outcome again and again. Along with education, more research needs to be done to figure out just how all the compounds interact and effect our endocannabinoid system, which helps regulate a lot of important functions in our body, like digestion, inflammation and mood.

"I hope to see more research and testing, so we can share it with the consumer," says Hadar. "It's something that we really try to promote here at Oregrown, and really educate our customers on what they're buying—because you want your customer to have a good experience so they come back. It's the only way we're going to survive as an industry."

JUST WHAT THE DOCTOR (HASN'T) ORDERED

Few physicians are schooled in CBD, so doctors and patients are finding new ways to learn how it can help.

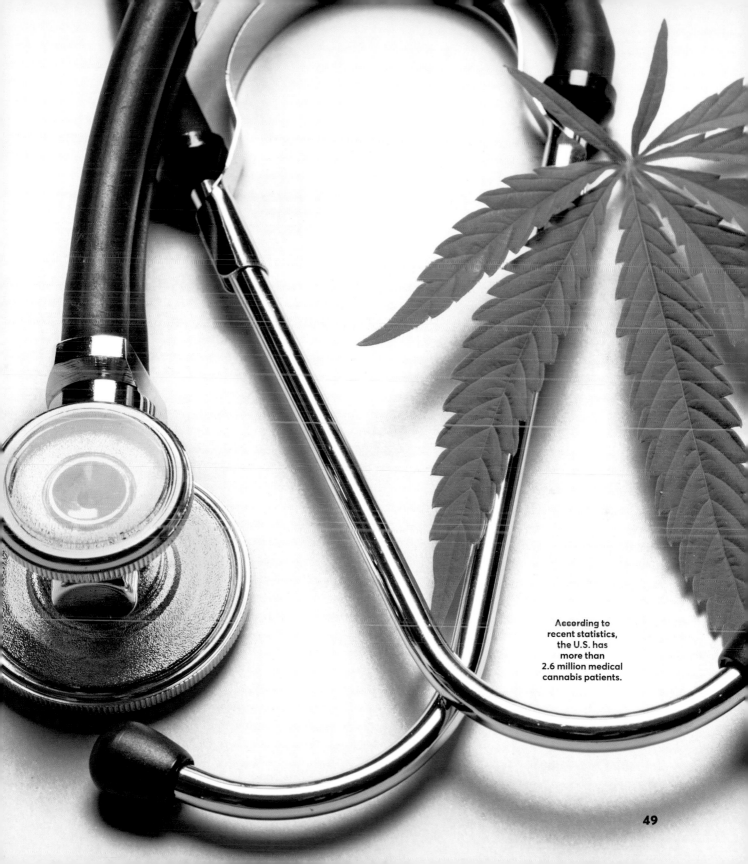

According to recent statistics, the U.S. has more than 2.6 million medical cannabis patients.

THE IDEA THAT CANNABIS can be a cure for most of what ails you is not exactly a new one. It's reportedly been used therapeutically for thousands of years, with ancient Persian texts touting its curative powers. However, it's only been in the past few years that U.S. health-care professionals started taking a serious interest in possibly suggesting medical marijuana to help their patients. Given how relatively new cannabis research is in this country—it only goes back a couple of decades—it shouldn't be too surprising that fewer than 15 percent of medical and nursing schools teach future health-care pros about the human endocannabinoid system and how it interacts with CBD.

Hence, "there's a knowledge gap within the medical community about CBD and how it can be used," says Anna Symonds, the director of education for East Fork Cultivars, a prominent Oregon cannabis farm that specializes in teaching cannabis professionals and consumers about the science of CBD. This means many medical practitioners aren't comfortable talking about CBD because they just don't have the information—and they don't want to simply guess. And patients who could be benefiting from cannabis aren't necessarily getting the best possible treatment.

■ Creating Collaborations

As CBD becomes increasingly popular, how can physicians learn enough in order to properly advise patients about its medical properties? Part of the solution is for them to do the same thing everyone else is doing: Pay attention to the articles and news pieces about CBD and study it in greater detail than non medical professionals.

"The more research that comes out on CBD, the more comfortable medical professionals will be using it therapeutically," says Symonds. "Practitioners are slowly becoming more interested in CBD and how it can be used in treatments."

Reading up on the research that's publicly available certainly helps make physicians more aware of what CBD can do, but for solid suggestions as to what patients should actually take, there needs to be something more. That's why in states that allow medical marijuana use, there's a trend toward official collaborations between medical practitioners and the cannabis industry. One leading example of this is Oregon Health and Science University, a teaching hospital in Portland, Oregon, that offers regular workshops on cannabis for clinical providers.

However, for those who don't have access to programs like OHSU's, there are other national groups that offer similar assistance for those in the medical field. That includes organizations such as the Cannabis Nurses Network, the International Cannabinoid Research

Society and medicalcannabisinstitute.org, which provide cannabis education courses geared toward health-care providers.

On the flip side, when it comes to patients seeking a health-care provider who is well-versed in CBD therapies, the process can be equally challenging. While some dispensaries have educated budtenders on staff, it's still a good idea to consult with a medical professional if at all possible. Since chances are not great that your doctor has been schooled in CBD, these patient resources may help.

• **The Society of Cannabis Clinicians** (cannabisclinicians.org) can help patients find local providers and clinicians who are taking continuing education courses to learn more about CBD.

• **The American Cannabis Nurses Association** (cannabisnurses.org), whose mission it is to advance excellence in cannabis nursing through advocacy, collaboration, education, research and policy development, provides a list of medical programs by state, as well as a collection of recommended reading for patients and nurses.

• **Projectcbd.org** gathers various medical studies that look at the benefits of CBD; **PubMed** (ncbi.nlm.nih.gov/pubmed) is an online government database of biomedical literature and journal articles.

• **Realm of Caring** (theroc.us) features a robust list of CBD providers that is organized by specialty and state, as well as a database of multiple medical cannabis studies. Says Courtney Collins, ROC's director of education, "We help if someone wants to look into CBD therapy but their health-care provider won't talk to them about it."

62%
Percentage of U.S. pharmacy schools that say they include medical marijuana in their curriculum.

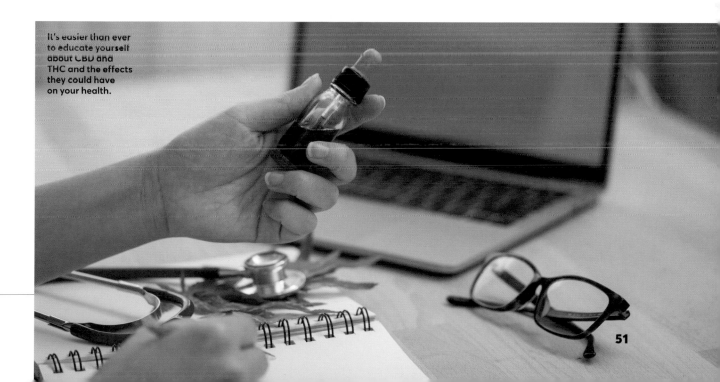

It's easier than ever to educate yourself about CBD and THC and the effects they could have on your health.

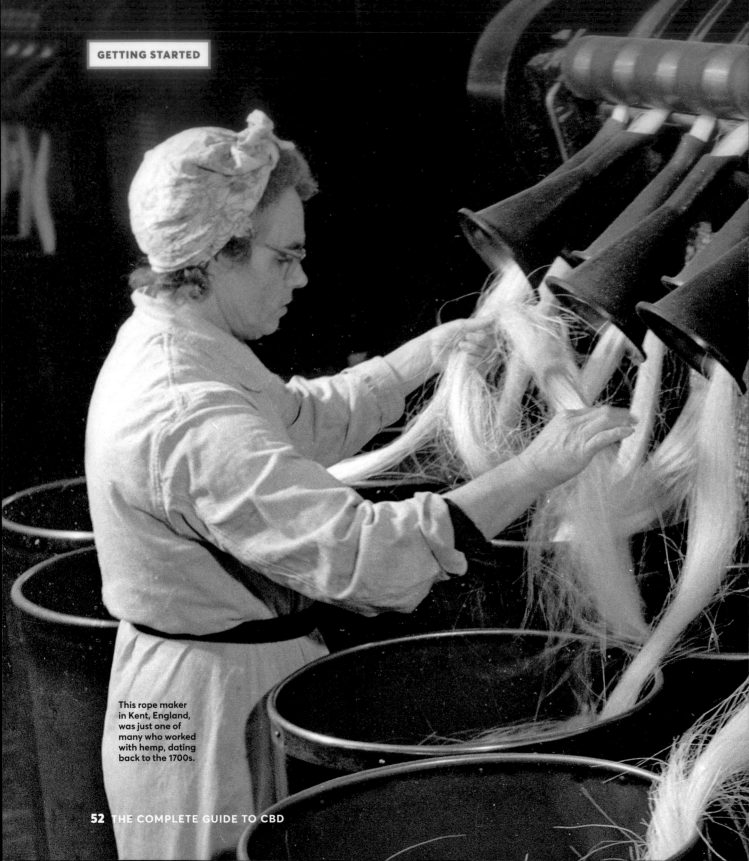

This rope maker in Kent, England, was just one of many who worked with hemp, dating back to the 1700s.

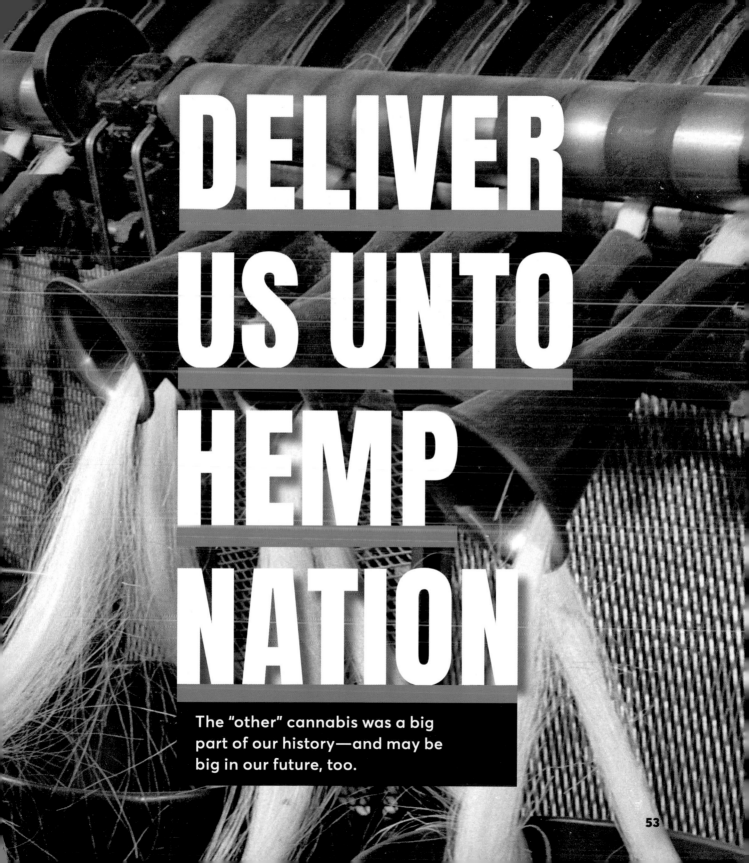

DELIVER US UNTO HEMP NATION

The "other" cannabis was a big part of our history—and may be big in our future, too.

THINK OF HEMP AND marijuana as the plant world's version of the soap opera's "evil twin" gimmick. You know in your heart that both are very much alike; but at the same time, one has developed a generous and helpful reputation while the other gets a bad rap as a problem child.

For centuries, hemp has proven invaluable in making everything from rope to paper to food. However, once the 20th century rolled around, the world took an intense dislike to the psychoactive qualities of its cannabis sativa cousin, marijuana. As a result, all forms of the cannabis plant fell out of favor.

"It's not really hard to get confused," explains David Rheins, founder and director of the Marijuana Business Association. "Just remember that both hemp and cannabis are part of the sativa plant. The difference is what you're breeding each for." Adds Morris Beegle, founder, president and CEO of We Are For Better Alternatives (WAFBA), "It's all cannabis. The only thing that makes it hemp versus marijuana is the percent of THC in the plant." As in, if it contains less than 0.3 percent of the psychoactive compound THC, it's hemp and can be tapped legally for its CBD, the healing property in cannabis.

To better understand where the plant came from and where it might be headed, here's a brief history of hemp.

■ In the Beginning

Hemp has been growing around the world since humanity decided to write down its history. (Which, ironically, would eventually be done using paper made from hemp.)

"What we do know about the plant is that it's been around since the dawn of civilization and we started to grow crops," explains Beegle, noting that the earliest appearance of hemp may have been 10,000 B.C. in Asia. "[People] used it to

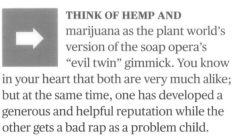

History of Hemp Time Line

10000 B.C.

The earliest evidence of hemp comes from rope imprints found on Chinese pottery created in this era.

10000 B.C.

make the early versions of sails and rope. It was also traditionally used for food, for fiber to make clothing and for building materials."

The first recorded use of the plant as medicine was in 2737 B.C., by Chinese emperor Shen Neng. Not too much later, Hindus referred to it as "sacred grass" and used it ritually as an offering to Shiva. By around possibly 300 B.C., the nomadic Scythian people were also instrumental in developing more spiritual uses for the hemp plant.

The first evidence of hemp-derived paper showed up in China around 100 B.C., and by 100 A.D., hemp rope was found in England and soon spread all across Europe. As practical as the plant was, though, it also managed to literally become a work of art. European painters like van Gogh and Rembrandt created their masterpieces on canvas. (The word canvas is derived from the Vulgar Latin cannabaceus, which means "made from

hemp.") That's a pretty classy turn of events for a plant that at one point grew out of control in so many places it would eventually be known as "ditch weed."

■ Coming to America

Hundreds of years before it became illegal to grow cannabis in America, it was actually illegal *not* to. The early American

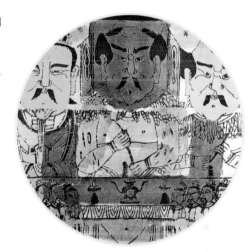

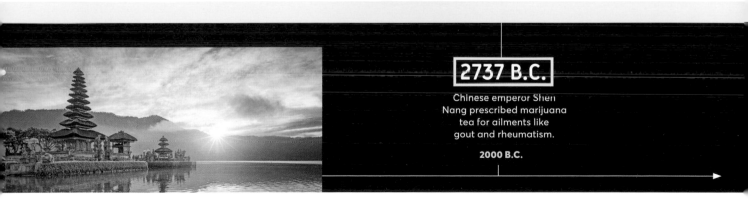

2737 B.C.

Chinese emperor Shen Nang prescribed marijuana tea for ailments like gout and rheumatism.

2000 B.C.

colonists were required by the British government to plant and cultivate hemp in order to keep its empire stocked with rope, sails and other essentials required when conquering the Western world.

Hemp was considered so important—not to mention profitable—that Founding Fathers like George Washington grew acres of it on their own land; Benjamin Franklin stocked his fledgling printing plant with hemp paper.

"The draft of the Declaration of Independence was on hemp. The first flag was made from hemp," says Lex Pelger, science director for Bluebird Botanicals, a Colorado-based manufacturer of hemp products. "It was like oil is today—a vital material, particularly in times of war."

By the late 1800s, parts of the hemp plant were still being used for goods like clothes, rope and paper, but the medicinal element had become even more popular. Cannabis was a part of all kinds of lotions, drinks and pills Americans could find at their neighborhood apothecary, and nobody seemed to mind.

■ The Tide Turns

In the beginning, hemp helped make the world a better place. However, when the 20th century rolled around, cannabis was something that tore the world apart. In the early 1900s, spurred on by alarmist stories about "marihuana" printed in the tabloids run by William Randolph Hearst, the plant was falsely derided as something

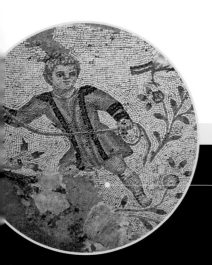

600 A.D.

European nations are regularly using hemp fibers for a variety of products.

300 A.D.

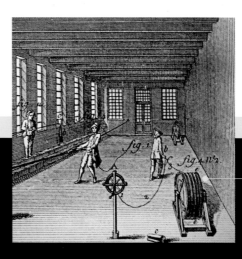

1700s–1900s

Mexican immigrants enjoyed before going on sadistic crime sprees. Even though U.S. Department of Agriculture scientists created paper in 1916 from a new, environmentally friendly form of hemp pulp, the conversation about cannabis had shifted. It didn't help that the DuPont Chemical Company, which was developing fibers like rayon and nylon, saw hemp as a threat because it was something people could grow themselves. The final blow to cannabis came when Congress passed the Marihuana Tax Act of 1937. This new law didn't ban sales of marijuana products outright, but it placed such a prohibitive tax on them that it might as well have.

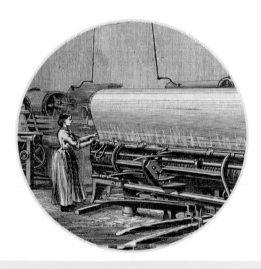

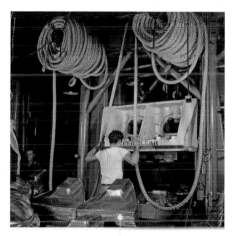

1750–1900

As colonists began growing hemp, factories in the United Kingdom used it to make items like rope and fishing nets.

1942

With the advent of World War II, hemp was used to make ropes that then helped in building parts for airplanes.

1940

> ## Industrial use of hemp got lumped in with marijuana use and it destroyed hemp around this country."
> —Morris Beegle, president, WAFBA

"Industrial use of hemp got lumped in with all that, and it destroyed hemp around this country," says Beegle.

Hemp still had plenty of supporters. In 1938, an article in *Popular Mechanics* claimed that it could become a major cash crop for the U.S. "Hemp is the standard fiber of the world," according to the story. "It can be used to produce

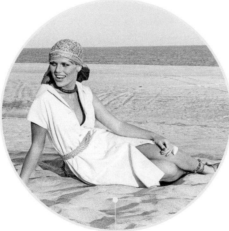

more than 25,000 products, ranging from dynamite to cellophane."

In 1942, the federal government realized that the country needed hemp because World War II had interrupted the flow of other industrial fibers to the U.S. The Tax Act was temporarily lifted, and the feds even produced a film, *Hemp for Victory*, praising the plant and encouraging American farmers to grow it to help the war effort. By 1943, there were 375,000 legal acres of it growing across the country.

This support didn't last long. After the war ended, so did government-approved hemp farming. By the 1960s, the primary image associated with cannabis was tie-dye-wearing hippies on college campuses, protesting the Vietnam War. Explains Rheins, "The hemp industry went out of its way to distance itself as marijuana was demonized. Hemp was seen as just an old-school thing. It wasn't demonized so much as it just wasn't in fashion."

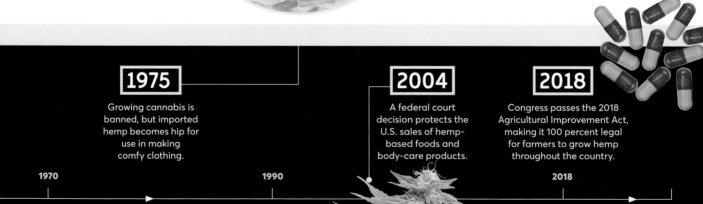

1975
Growing cannabis is banned, but imported hemp becomes hip for use in making comfy clothing.

2004
A federal court decision protects the U.S. sales of hemp-based foods and body-care products.

2018
Congress passes the 2018 Agricultural Improvement Act, making it 100 percent legal for farmers to grow hemp throughout the country.

1970

1990

2018

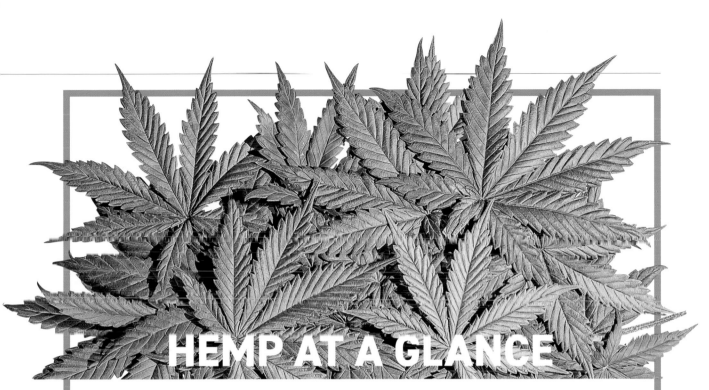

HEMP AT A GLANCE

■ In 2018 the Drug Enforcement Administration (DEA) changed the definition of marijuana to exclude hemp; the plant is no longer considered a controlled substance.

■ The decision means that hemp—including hemp plants and hemp-derived CBD products at or below the 0.3 percent THC threshold—no longer requires DEA registration.

■ The DEA guidance gives financial institutions more confidence in doing business with hemp companies. Some banks had shied away from doing business over this lack of clarity.

■ The U.S. Food and Drug Administration (FDA) is also reworking rules governing cosmetics, dietary supplements, food additives and food. The U.S. Hemp Industries Association has advised the FDA that the existing rules for those products should be expanded to embrace hemp extracts.

THE SHIFT The 2018 Farm Bill changed federal policy regarding hemp, removing it from the Controlled Substances Act. Hemp is now considered an agricultural product. The bill legalized hemp (under certain restrictions) and expanded the definition of hemp from the last Farm Bill (2014). The bill also allows states and tribes to submit a plan and apply for primary regulatory authority over the production of hemp in their state or in their tribal territory. A state plan must include certain requirements, such as keeping track of land, testing methods and disposal of plants or products that exceed the allowed THC concentration (above 0.3 percent).

State policy makers have addressed various policy issues, including the definition of hemp, licensure of growers, regulation and certification of seeds, and the establishment of state-wide commissions and the legal protection of growers. At least 47 states have enacted legislation to establish hemp-cultivation and production programs.

Every state—except Idaho, South Dakota and Missouri—allows cultivation of hemp for commercial, research or pilot programs.

Source: National Conference of State Legislatures

2

HELPING WITH HEALING

IT MAY NOT BE A CURE-ALL, BUT PLENTY OF PATIENTS OUT THERE NOW CONSIDER CBD TO BE AT LEAST A "CURE-A-LOT." FROM CANCER TO STRESS TO SPORTS INJURIES, THE LIST OF ISSUES IT CAN POTENTIALLY HELP WITH CONTINUES TO GROW.

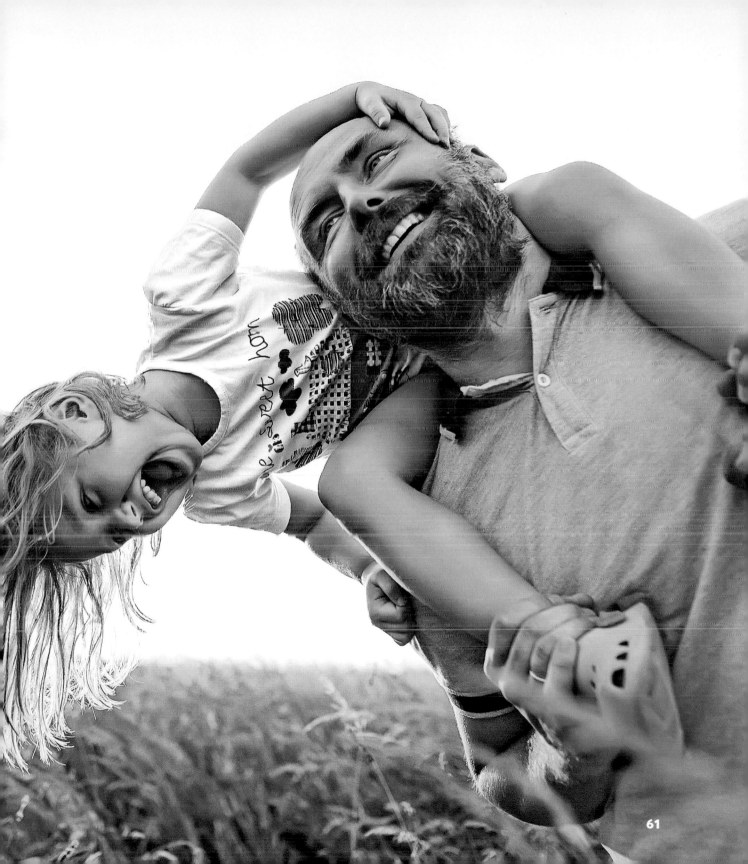

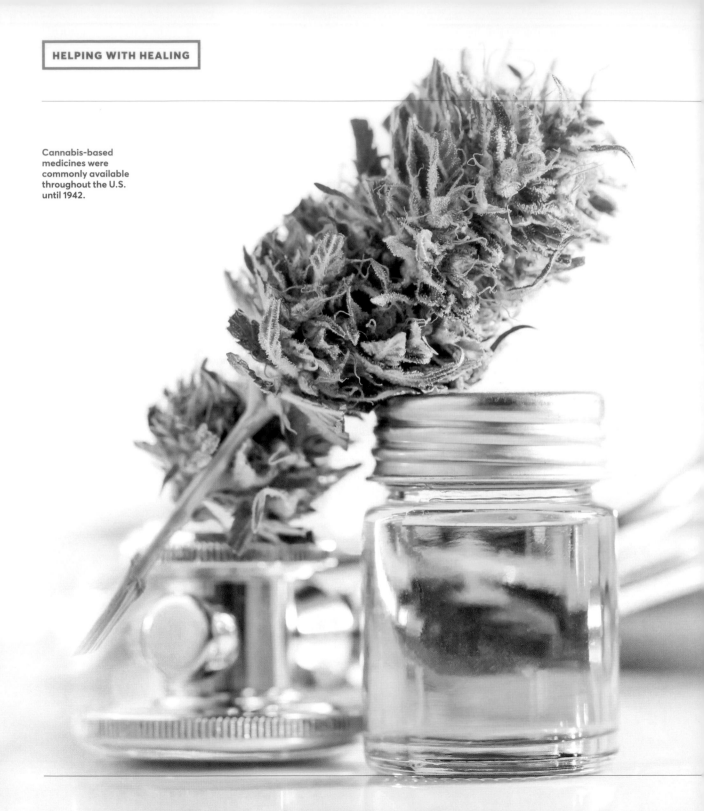

Cannabis-based medicines were commonly available throughout the U.S. until 1942.

A-Z CANNABIS

GUIDE TO HEALING

From Alzheimer's to Zoster, this comprehensive list looks at a variety of ailments and what, if any, relief cannabis can help provide.

NO MATTER WHERE WE'RE from, who we voted for or how we felt about the *Game of Thrones* finale, there are two things pretty much all of us have in common. First, at some point in our lives, we're going to get sick. And second, we've recently read about, or discussed with someone, the medicinal potential of marijuana. Cannabis has started to seem like a miracle drug, the cure for whatever ails us. Americans have come to believe so much in the reported healing powers of this plant that one poll found that more than 90 percent of adults want medical marijuana legalized on the federal level.

Still, solid research is not easy to come by. It can be difficult to separate fact from fiction when it comes to determining what marijuana can help with. So, we spoke to cannabis experts Emma Chasen, Mary Brown, Dr. Bonni Goldstein and Dr. Mary Clifton to get their thoughts on the conditions for which this plant might provide relief.

Cannabis Experts

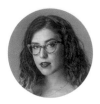

EMMA CHASEN

A graduate of Brown University with a degree in medicinal plant research, Chasen has worked as general manager and director of education for the popular Portland, Oregon, dispensary Farma. She now operates Eminent Consulting, which offers cannabis education for those in the industry as well as for medical and recreational users.

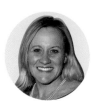

MARY BROWN

Brown works as the executive director and lead consultant for the Seattle-based SMJ Consulting at the AIMS Institute, which offers medical patients education services and individualized wellness programs that are centered on cannabinoid therapy.

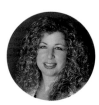

DR. BONNI GOLDSTEIN

The former chief resident at Children's Hospital Los Angeles, she is now the director of the California-based Canna-Centers, a wellness organization that educates patients on the use of cannabis for serious and chronic conditions. Goldstein is also the author of the book *Cannabis Revealed*.

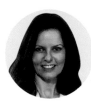

DR. MARY CLIFTON

CBD and cannabis expert Clifton is an internal medicine doctor with more than 20 years of experience. She is now a leading voice in telemedicine, and offers consultations through her website, cbdandcannabisinfo.com. Clifton is also the author of *The Grass Is Greener: Medical Marijuana, THC & CBD Oil: Reversing Chronic Pain, Inflammation and Disease*.

Research is focusing on the role cannabinoids may play in reducing dementia.

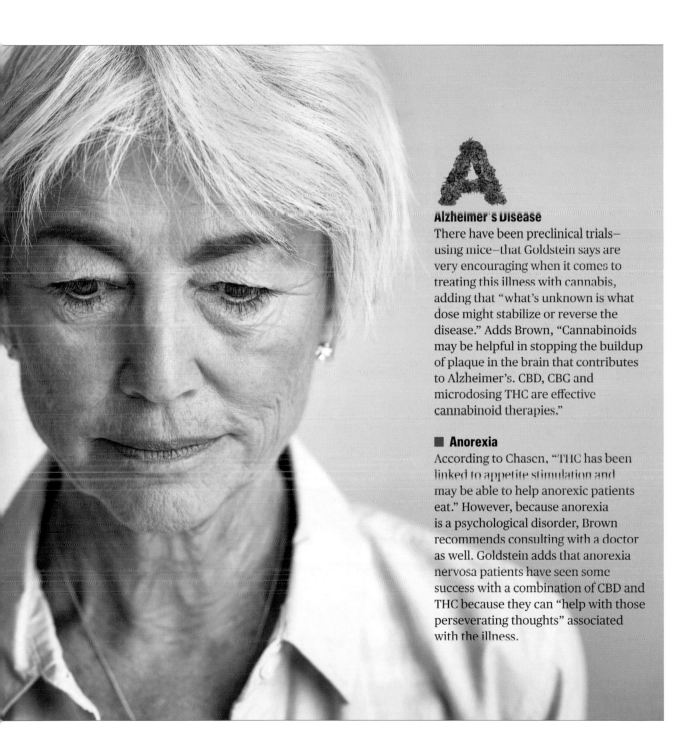

A

Alzheimer's Disease

There have been preclinical trials—using mice—that Goldstein says are very encouraging when it comes to treating this illness with cannabis, adding that "what's unknown is what dose might stabilize or reverse the disease." Adds Brown, "Cannabinoids may be helpful in stopping the buildup of plaque in the brain that contributes to Alzheimer's. CBD, CBG and microdosing THC are effective cannabinoid therapies."

■ Anorexia

According to Chasen, "THC has been linked to appetite stimulation and may be able to help anorexic patients eat." However, because anorexia is a psychological disorder, Brown recommends consulting with a doctor as well. Goldstein adds that anorexia nervosa patients have seen some success with a combination of CBD and THC because they can "help with those perseverating thoughts" associated with the illness.

■ Anxiety

CBD, as well as the cannabinoid CBG, have shown potential in helping to treat anxiety, explains Brown. But it's a tricky situation. On the one hand, Clifton says there has been at least one significant study that indicated some cannabis could improve the symptoms of anxiety. On the other, she notes that "you can sometimes aggravate [your anxiety] with a high-THC product or create a little paranoia."

Back Pain

The experts all agree that when it comes to easing chronic pain, CBD in particular can be very effective. And with the "entourage effect" that comes from throwing in other cannabinoids, "it could probably do even better," says Clifton. There's also the analgesic (muscle relaxing) properties of cannabis that Brown says can bring relief, with Chasen noting that the use of topical medicines is best, because they can be applied right to the point of pain.

Common Cold

As great as it would be to finally have a cure for the common cold, we'll have to wait a bit longer because, says Clifton, there's been no significant research into whether cannabis can help. However, as with other herbal treatments, she does say that "there is definitely immunity modulation that goes on [with cannabis] that probably helps reduce the intensity of the symptoms if you're taking it before you get sick."

■ Crohn's Disease ▶

Thanks to the multitude of CB2 receptors in the lower abdominal organs, according to Brown, the cannabinoids CBD and CBG could help ease the pain of Crohn's, particularly when consumed orally. Goldstein suggests using some degree of THC as well. Explains Chasen, "So many cannabis compounds can help calm the smooth muscle of the digestive system and help Crohn's patients more effectively manage their disease."

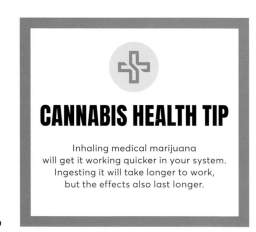

CANNABIS HEALTH TIP

Inhaling medical marijuana
will get it working quicker in your system.
Ingesting it will take longer to work,
but the effects also last longer.

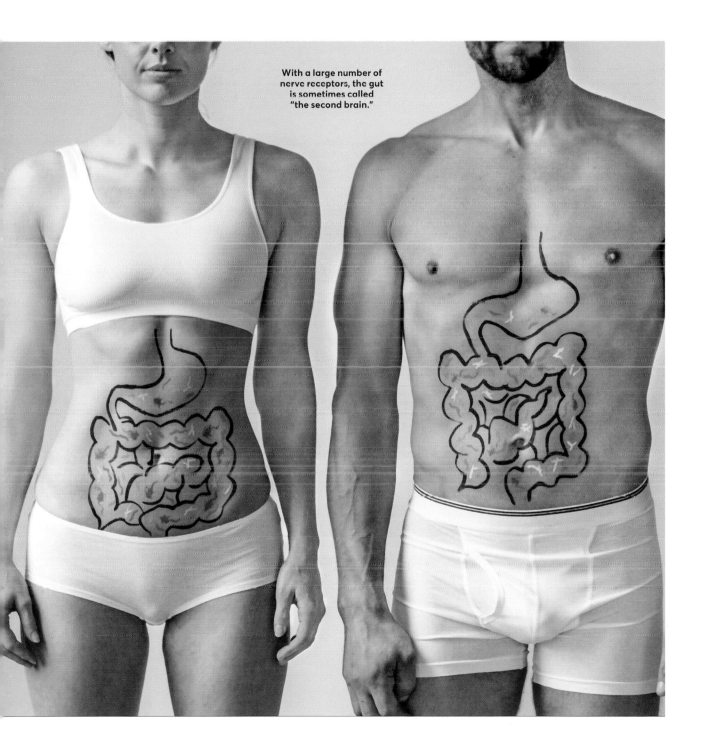

With a large number of nerve receptors, the gut is sometimes called "the second brain."

67

Depression

"You'll probably see some benefit with THC and CBD, although there's less data on this than there is for anxiety," explains Clifton. They may work because the compounds within cannabis, adds Chasen, interact with our serotonin and dopamine systems, which modulate our mood. "CBD is a great low-risk option, especially when coupled with terpenes such as limonene and b-caryophyllene," she says. "THC may also be helpful. However, it can also heighten depressive symptoms if used in too high a concentration. Therefore, keep it low and go for something CBD-dominant."

■ Diabetes

While there's no concrete proof that cannabis can cure this illness in humans, Goldstein says there has been a preclinical trial that looked into stopping type 1 diabetes with lab mice. The result? "They found that if they started CBD very early on after mice developed diabetes, they could reverse it," she explains. What cannabis can do for people, though, is help ease the pain of diabetes' side effects, such as retinal damage, diabetic neuropathy and nerve pain. In addition, she adds that it can have a positive effect on balancing the body's sugars, but it's also critical to eat better and exercise more, too, rather than just relying on cannabis alone.

Epilepsy

This is one condition that has been extensively studied, to the point where there's even an FDA-approved, cannabis-derived drug to help with seizures: Epidiolex. "High-CBD strains have been reported to greatly reduce seizure frequency, and THC has been included in reports as having potential for rescue during seizures," says Brown. While Clifton is encouraged by studies she's seen supporting this conclusion, she also cautions that the dosage required is "in the hundreds of milligrams."

Fibromyalgia

The anti-inflammatory and pain-mediation properties of cannabis make it a strong option for fibromyalgia sufferers. Brown cites a study of 390 participants with the illness where 62 percent reported cannabis as "very effective" in treating their symptoms and 33 percent reported that it helped "a little." As for what to take, she says that "the ratio of CBD to THC that benefits patients is based on individual preference."

CBD-infused teas are popular for flu symptoms caused by inflammation, like sore throats.

▼ Flu

It's the same situation as with colds, according to Clifton. Cannabis can potentially help with "immune system response modulation"—meaning for it to do any good, you need to be using it already to help your body fight off the virus that can give you the flu. "There's no hard evidence that shows using cannabis while ill will make you get well quicker or block the severity of the illness," explains Goldstein, adding that it can help flu sufferers sleep, lose some of their achiness and get their appetite back.

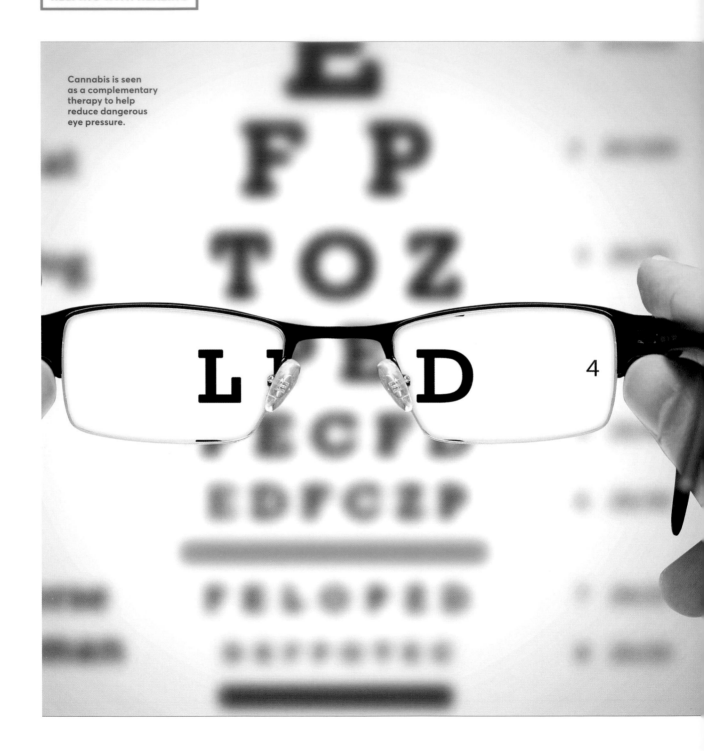

Cannabis is seen as a complementary therapy to help reduce dangerous eye pressure.

◀ Glaucoma

We've known since the release of a study in 1971 that smoking cannabis can possibly ease eye pressure and help glaucoma sufferers. "Through its analgesic and anti-inflammatory properties, cannabis can be used as a pain reliever and may reduce swelling of the optic nerve," says Brown. However, Goldstein cautions that "despite the fact that it's on every state [medical program] list of what can be approved for glaucoma, cannabis isn't mono therapy." Instead, it should be seen as "an adjunct" to other treatments recommended by your doctor. Chasen suggests the daily oral ingestion of THC may relieve pressure around the eye, but Goldstein notes that "CBD has been shown to elevate interocular pressure, so you have to be very careful. There needs to be more research in this realm."

Hepatitis

Because this condition results from having an inflamed liver, Clifton believes that cannabis can "have a proactive effect" if taken in low doses.

Insomnia

"Cannabis can act as an effective support for insomnia patients," says Brown. "CBN is a complementary cannabinoid to THC and CBD for enhancing the sleep-inducing effects." Chasen enthusiastically concurs. "THC and CBD can both help regulate sleep cycling, though THC may keep you out of REM sleep," she explains. "Therefore, opt for a higher concentration of CBD compared to THC. Plus, terpenes like linalool can really help get you to sleep–and help you stay asleep!"

Jock Itch

This isn't a job for cannabis or CBD directly, according to Clifton. However, using a compound such as pinene or limonene that's included in a topical such as a salve or lotion can have an antibacterial effect, which may not only ease jock itch but also outbreaks of things like toe fungus.

Kidney Disease

Cannabinoids like THC and CBD are able to pass through the kidney's filtration system but stop to interact with the cannabinoid receptors that regulate kidney function. THC also appears to help manage chronic pain among patients with chronic kidney disease, according to a study published in the *Canadian Journal of Kidney Health and Disease,* which found patients who were treated with nonsynthetic cannabinoids were up to three times more likely to report at least a 30 percent reduction in chronic neuropathic pain compared with a placebo.

Lupus

This is another case of cannabis possibly helping with the symptoms of the condition, if not the condition itself. "Cannabis can help relieve pain and inflammation common in patients with lupus," says Brown. "It is possible that cannabinoids can act as an immuno-suppressant, which is beneficial to combat the hyperactive immune system that accompanies [the condition]."

Menstrual Cramps

Depending on the source of the cramps, Brown notes, a treatment that includes a combination of high CBD and broad-spectrum low THC could help to ease the cramping pain. Meanwhile, Chasen suggests the use of vaginal suppositories with a 1:1 CBD to THC ratio, although "consuming through other routes of administration, like oral or inhalation, may also be helpful."

▶ Migraines

Hormonal migraines "are best targeted with CBD:CBG," according to Brown. "THC can sometimes make the condition worse. If migraines are caused from stress, then THC:CBD may be a good combination."

Multiple Sclerosis

When it comes to neurodegenerative diseases like multiple sclerosis, CBD and CBG are apparently "showing promise in slowing the progression" of those conditions, Brown explains. In addition, "reduction in anxiety and improved sleep are commonly reported with cannabis use amongst MS patients."

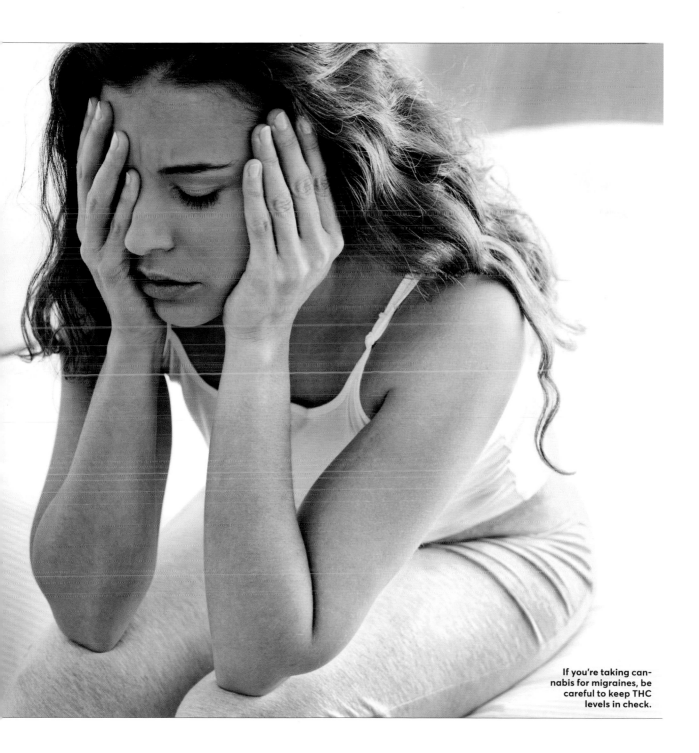

If you're taking can-
nabis for migraines, be
careful to keep THC
levels in check.

Nausea

"This is one of the few ailments cannabis can conclusively help with," says Chasen. Whether it's dealing with the loss of appetite in HIV/AIDS patients or the aftereffects of chemotherapy, cannabis is now viewed by many as a legitimate form of relief due to the way it can ease nausea. "Inhaled cannabis rich in THC, CBD and THC8 can offer immediate relief of nausea from various causes," says Brown. This is why Clifton credits cannabis with being a significant factor for the decline in deaths from HIV/AIDS.

Obesity

Ironically, while experts believe cannabis can help increase appetite for those suffering from anorexia or the aftereffects of chemotherapy, it might also be able to help curb obesity. Says Chasen, "THC, CBD and limonene...have shown anorexic effects and may be able to reduce appetite." Adds Brown, "Cannabinoids can help regulate the human system. Preclinical studies demonstrate that THCV can act as an appetite suppressant, so strains rich in it are great to avoid the common 'munchies' side effect of cannabis use."

Parkinson's Disease

The good news is that there has been a lot of information gathered about the relationship between cannabis and Parkinson's, according to Clifton. The not-so-good news? Clifton says that in half of the cases studied, cannabis didn't help slow the tremors associated with the condition. Meanwhile, Chasen suggests that FECO–a full-spectrum alcohol preparation with a high concentration of CBD–"may be able to dramatically reduce tremors." Either way, don't dismiss cannabis as a way to help. "Even in situations where the tremors weren't reduced, patients reported an improvement in symptoms," Clifton says. "They think it's because cannabis manages the anxiety and sleep disorders around Parkinson's." Brown adds that "the entourage effect of cannabinoids, specifically those high in CBG, can help to diminish neurodegeneration. Often, patients are finding reduction in spasticity with inhaled cannabis."

■ Psoriasis

This is something that Clifton says she takes personally because "I have horrible skin. It was almost too much to live in when I was younger, and I had a standing appointment once a month with dermatologists." CBD in the form of topicals has definitely provided relief. In addition, according to Brown, "oral administration of full-spectrum cannabis, including CBD:THC:CBC, has shown tremendous potential in reducing the frequent flare-ups psoriasis patients experience."

Q Fever ▼

According to the Mayo Clinic, this is a bacteria-driven infection that causes flu-like symptoms and can be transmitted to humans through animals, particularly barnyard animals like goats, cows and sheep. At this time, there is no direct research delving into how cannabis use might provide a cure for Q Fever. However, as is the case with the flu, using it might improve your immune system enough to fight off an infection or ease some of the symptoms of Q Fever, such as headaches, muscle aches, fatigue and nausea.

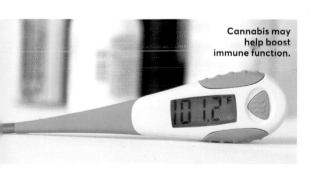

Cannabis may help boost immune function.

Rheumatoid Arthritis

"Because arthritis patients have a higher amount of CB2 receptors in their joints, high CBD:THC ratios such as 30:1 in oral form may offer relief," says Brown. However, don't see cannabis as the only thing you need to add to relieve arthritis pain. Explains Clifton, "Inflammation comes from the inside out," so if you have a poor diet and have been storing up unhealthy fat or you're sleeping less, you leave yourself open to other health problems that can exacerbate your joint aches.

Stroke

There may well be plenty of help to be had here. Brown points out that "cannabinoids are neuroprotective," meaning that the antioxidant properties of CBD and CBG have been "observed to potentially slow brain damage in the aftermath of a stroke that is mostly associated with the increased level of oxidative stress, excitotoxity and inflammation." Plus, she adds, the anti-inflammatory properties of THC "show promise" when it comes to stroke recovery.

Tourette's Syndrome

Brown and Clifton both cite studies done in Germany on the effect of cannabis on children with Tourette's. While the results seem to indicate that THC "could increase obsessive-compulsive disorder behavioral tendencies" that are often associated with Tourette's, says Brown, "high CBD and low THC—20:1—would be the recommendation" for possible treatment. Clifton does say that in one German study, one child's Tourette's got inexplicably worse while using cannabis. However, "they circled back and it turned out he'd quit using it and was using alcohol to control his symptoms. As soon as he stopped using that and began using cannabis again, he got better."

Vascular Disease

While research in humans is still in progress, animal studies have shown that CBD may help protect against vascular damage caused by a diet that's high in glucose. It's also been shown to have a direct impact on isolated arteries, helping to reduce vascular tension when administered in animal models. And CBD's anti-inflammatory properties may play a role in reducing tissue damage that can occur after a period of ischemia (lack of oxygen to the heart). While researchers caution that more studies are necessary, investigators say it appears that CBD plays a positive role in treatment that supports the peripheral and cerebral vasculature.

Ulcerative Colitis

Not unlike Crohn's disease and other conditions involving the stomach, there is the possibility of pain relief from cannabis for sufferers of ulcerative colitis. There are "abundant CB2 receptors in the lower abdominal organs," explains Brown, and they can potentially respond very well to a treatment involving a combination of CBD and CBG.

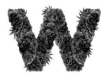

Wasting Syndrome

Also called "cachexia," this is a symptom of many chronic conditions such as HIV/AIDS, chronic renal failure, multiple sclerosis and cancer. It causes extreme weight loss and the wasting away of muscles. Brown says that there have been cases where THC and THC8 have been used to combat cachexia.

Fragile X Syndrome

Many children who are diagnosed with fragile X syndrome a genetic condition that causes a range of developmental problems—also experience behavioral issues like anxiety, hyperactive behavior, attention deficit disorder and autism spectrum disorder. Early research indicates that a pharmaceutical CBD gel from Zynerba Pharmaceuticals may significantly improve behavioral symptoms in children and adolescents with the syndrome.

Yeast Infection

Similar to the situation with jock itch, according to Clifton, using a medicine that contains pinenes may take care of the inflammation that leads to yeast infections. Brown also says that "there is a possibility of CBD and CBG showing promise due to their antifungal and antibacterial properties. This does not include the inhalation mode."

Zoster

This virus, known to cause shingles as well as chicken pox, can cause serious pain. It can be notoriously difficult to treat, according to Clifton, but cannabis can potentially modulate the agony because it is what she refers to as "neuropathic." "I would take something orally, a product containing THC, because it can work deep in the tissue" where inflammation is occurring, she advises.

A vaccine can help protect against shingles.

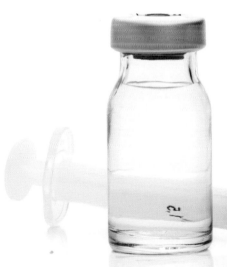

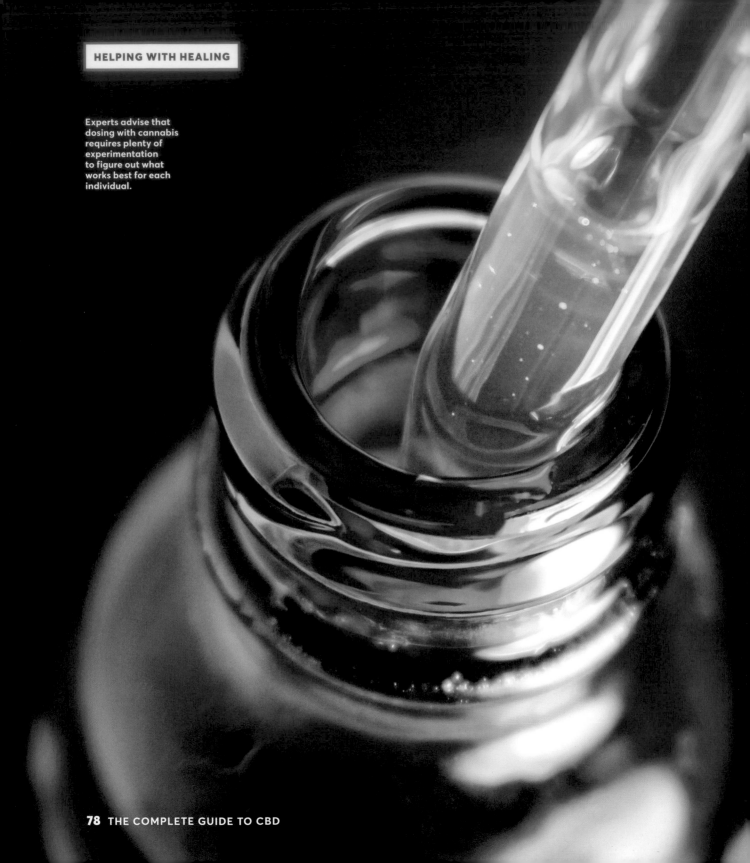

Experts advise that dosing with cannabis requires plenty of experimentation to figure out what works best for each individual.

How Much Do You Need?

Before trying CBD for the first time, it's a good Idea to follow these critical tips to determine your dose.

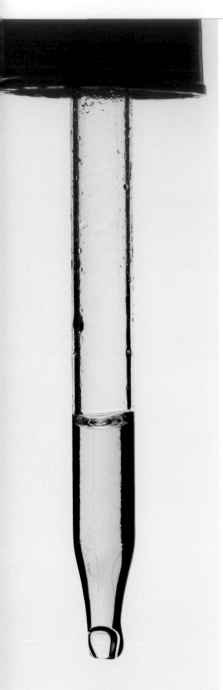

WHEN IT COMES TO finding the right CBD dosage for individual patients, experts agree that the only thing we know is that we don't know much.

"Determining the appropriate dosage is completely personal, and that's where confusion comes into the process," explains Zoe Sigman, program director for Project CBD, a national nonprofit cannabis-education group. "It all depends on who you are and what you need it for."

With prescription medicines, the process is simple: Go to your doctor. Tell him/her what's wrong. Get pills. Go home. With CBD, though, there is no standard dosing amount or procedure, so it can take a lot of trial and error before finding the relief you seek. With that in mind, we asked some industry experts to create this checklist for getting started.

1

Wonder Why

This may seem self-evident, but it's still the ideal starting point for any CBD journey. Decide precisely what you want to get out of the experience before it begins. "Before I consume a product, I check in with myself to ask, 'Why am I doing this?'" says Sigman. "'What am I hoping this will do?' That will establish a baseline to start from."

2

Check Your Expectations

Despite all the news stories and headlines saying otherwise, CBD is not a cure-all. "Moderate your expectations about what it can do," explains Jim Walsh, a public relations strategist who works with major cannabis brands like Bloom Farms. "I've heard people say, 'I took CBD and didn't notice any difference.' But your body needs to build up to it. Take it for at least a week to see how you feel."

3

Start Low and Go Slow

Since everybody is different, there is no one-dose-fits-all recommendation, so it's critical to begin with a small amount of CBD and gradually work your way up until you get the effect you are after. "This is to help facilitate your own understanding of your unique tolerances and sensitivities," says Charles McElroy, founder of Goldleaf, which makes dosing journals for cannabis patients.

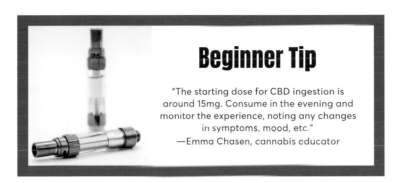

Beginner Tip

"The starting dose for CBD ingestion is around 15mg. Consume in the evening and monitor the experience, noting any changes in symptoms, mood, etc."
—Emma Chasen, cannabis educator

4
Have No Fear

Because CBD is nontoxic, new users shouldn't worry about taking too much since there are "almost no negative side effects," according to Sigman. "The risk of something bad happening is very low." While she doesn't recommend taking anything less than 5mg ("which doesn't seem like it would do much"), working up to 15mg or even 30mg would be fine, as long as you give it enough time to work—which could be days or even weeks.

5
Find Full Spectrum

This means looking for products that "aren't just CBD. They should have as many active compounds [from the cannabis plant] as possible," says Sigman. She cites research from Spain and Israel suggesting all these compounds work better together—aka the entourage effect—than when you just take an extracted dose of CBD.

6
Check the Test

Before you buy anything, says Sigman, check that the product has been tested at a third-party laboratory. "Make sure of the level of cannabinoids in it, the batch size it comes from, when it was created…. If you don't have those test results, you don't know what you're taking." And if the dispensary or website you're buying from says it doesn't have that information, keep looking until another retailer can provide it.

7
Make a Note

As you experiment with different doses of CBD, "keeping detailed notes about your CBD trials will help you understand what has worked best, what times of day you used it and the specifics of what the product was," says McElroy. This process literally puts down in black and white the information you'll need if you proceed with CBD treatments and eventually heal yourself.

FAMILY FRIENDLY

CBD may be the key when it comes to becoming a better parent.

A recent survey found that one in five parents uses cannabis, and 63 percent of those do so daily.

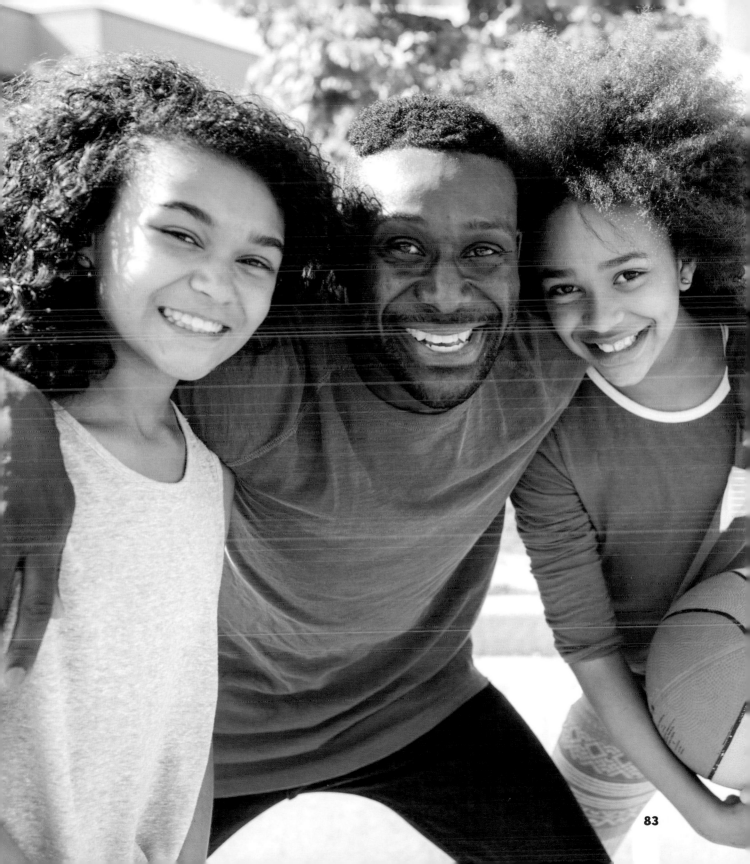

THERE WAS A TIME NOT THAT long ago when, if you wanted to be a good parent, you warned your kids against using cannabis. These days, however, you may find using it yourself makes you a better parent—at least when it comes to CBD.

It's not unlike taking a plane trip with your small children, according to Shira Adler, author of *The ABCs of CBD: The Essential Guide for Parents (And Regular Folks Too)* and founder of the health and wellness company Synergy by Shira Adler. "They instruct you to put on your own mask first in the case of an emergency, then take care of someone else," she says, adding that the same principle is true in our daily lives—except that instead of masks, "we should start with doing what we have to in order to have a decent day." In other words, if you want to take the best care of your kids, start by taking the best care of yourself. And CBD is as good a place to begin as any.

"I do think it's a good idea to use CBD to specifically help with parenting," explains cannabis industry educator and consultant Emma Chasen. "Parenting a child comes with a lot of stress, and CBD can be effective in managing and relieving it. It can be incredibly helpful, as it can be relaxing and also improve mood, while still allowing for heightened presence and focus. When a parent isn't in a state of high stress, CBD allows him or her to be more engaged with and enjoy their children."

Providing a Healthy Option

If you ask any parents how they're feeling, odds are the conversation will probably begin and end with a discussion of how exhausted they are. Let's face it: This is a job with pretty lousy hours, so it's easy to wear down quickly and completely. Meanwhile, the time-honored parental remedies for unwinding—wine, prescription medicines and, well, more wine—are not the healthiest options available. This is another area where CBD can help pooped parents: It can actually heal your body while also soothing it.

"Not only can CBD help parents relax, but—thanks to its antioxidant properties—it may help protect our cells from stress damage," says Jessie Gill, a cannabis nurse who also runs the educational website marijuanamommy.com. "When we experience stress, our cells create free radicals, which have negative effects on every area of our body. CBD may help whisk free radicals away, lessening the negative effects of stress on our bodies."

She adds that many of the parents she speaks to have reported an improvement in the quality and quantity of sleep, making all those two-hour drives to soccer tournaments less nerve-racking. Chasen adds that rather than seeing cannabis use as a sign of weakness, many moms are discovering it can be a sign of strength.

"There's Nothing to Hide"

"There are great groups here in Oregon that discuss cannabis and parenting,"

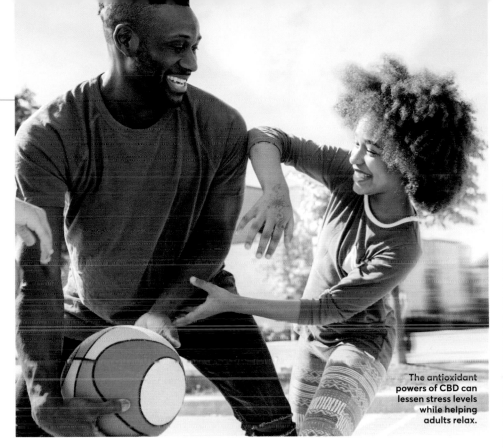

The antioxidant powers of CBD can lessen stress levels while helping adults relax.

Chasen says. "The organization Tokeativity has an ongoing event series—Canna Mamas—that employs education and community support to help moms feel empowered in their cannabis use."

She also recommends splimm.com, an online pot and parenting newsletter that describes itself as "the premier media outlet for families whose lives have been enhanced by cannabis." For those who want to see if CBD can enhance their mood, and therefore their parenting skills, Chasen has two important pieces of advice. First, make sure that the product they're using "doesn't look like candy and comes in childproof packaging." And second, be open and honest about what you're doing.

Whereas previous generations of parents tried to scare their children away from any sort of drug use, they were also less than forthright when it came to their own coping mechanisms. For too long, explains Adler, "moms could pop a Xanax or put liquor in sippy cups they'd sneak shots of at their kids' soccer games," but there was still "this stigma about having a joint."

"There is nothing to hide [with using CBD]," adds Chasen. "Hiding it implies that you're doing something wrong—and you're not. Talk to your kids about CBD in a rational way. Kids are smart. Explain to them that this is a medicine for grown-ups and kids who are really sick."

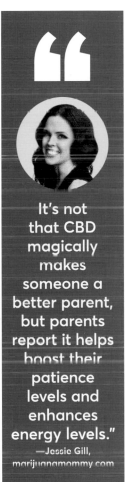

"It's not that CBD magically makes someone a better parent, but parents report it helps boost their patience levels and enhances energy levels."
—Jessie Gill, marijuanamommy.com

STOPPING THE STRESS

Anxiety sufferers are finding that CBD can help put them at ease.

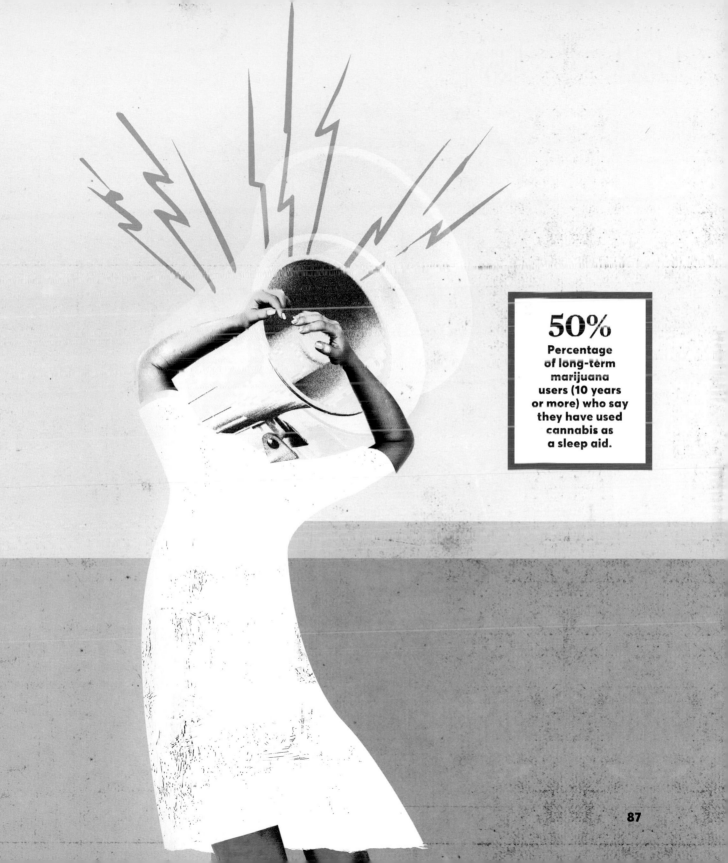

50%
Percentage
of long-term
marijuana
users (10 years
or more) who say
they have used
cannabis as
a sleep aid.

AT FIRST, THE IDEA OF USING cannabis as a way to treat anxiety seems counterintuitive. After all, as the stereotype goes, paranoia and anxiousness are potential side effects from using marijuana. However, as it turns out, while the THC in weed might cause those symptoms, the CBD is actually a great tool to curb them.

Take it from neuroscientist Michele Ross, who has studied the human endocannabinoid system and brain neurotransmitters for a decade. After years of suffering from anxiety, she found success balancing her moods with a CBD regimen.

She's far from alone when it comes to her situation. Anxiety disorders are the most common mental illness in the U.S., affecting 40 million adults. There hasn't been a lot of research to determine exactly how CBD can help, but one recent study of adults with PTSD found that within a month of starting to use it, nearly 80 percent reported a drop in anxiety levels, while 67 percent reported an improvement in their sleep.

As eager as Ross was to find relief from her anxiety, she was initially reluctant to try any sort of alternative medicine.

"Back in my college days, I was on anti-anxiety drugs because I had a lot of social anxiety," explains Ross. That condition only got worse in 2009, when she was a "houseguest" on the 11th season of CBS' reality series *Big Brother*.

"I ended up dealing with a lot of people, and I was definitely freaked out."

Although she was curious about all she was hearing about the purported benefits of CBD, Ross chose not to experiment with cannabis because she was still working in academia and didn't want to be associated with the stigma that still lingered around the plant.

"When you're a drug addiction scientist, you don't end up working with cannabis or CBD because they're still considered Schedule 1 drugs, so you can really mess up your career," she says. Instead, she put her experimentation with cannabis on hold until a few years later, when she left the academic world. At that point, she recalls, she was in her 30s and started using it because she also suffered from chronic pain and fibromyalgia and figured the THC in pot would take care of the problem.

"I had a lot of issues with using THC," she recalls. "Five milligrams of THC is considered a normal dose that people say won't get you anxious or too high. But no matter what dose of THC I use, there are two outcomes –I either fall asleep or I'm too high and paranoid. I've never been able to use THC effectively."

■ **Unexpected Benefits**

So Ross turned to CBD, since it was already well-chronicled as a way to treat chronic pain. What she

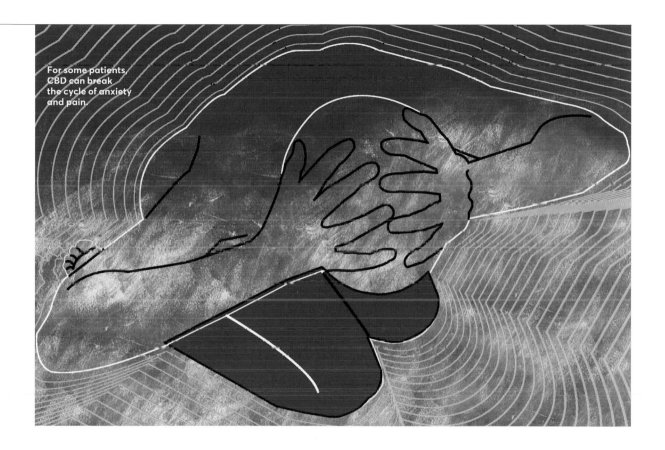

For some patients, CBD can break the cycle of anxiety and pain.

didn't realize was that pain and anxiety often go hand in hand—so suddenly, she had a medicine that could take care of two debilitating illnesses instead of just one. Clinical studies have shown that CBD interacts specifically with our bodies' serotonin receptors, known as (5-HT), the neurotransmitters that influence both pain and anxiety. Its effect on pain is understood to be mostly as an anti-inflammatory, while it benefits anxiety sufferers by stimulating feelings of relaxation and euphoria.

"I use CBD drops throughout the day just to help me relax, and I use them for my neck pain," says Ross. "When you have chronic pain you also have more anxiety. It's like you're trapped in this pain cycle–'I hurt! This sucks! And now I'm anxious about hurting more.' The CBD helps my muscles relax and it helps me focus."

One common mistake those looking to treat their anxiety with CBD may be making, though, is relying on a dosage that is too low to actually make an that is too low to actually make an impact. "CBD does reduce anxiety, but in high doses," Ross explains.

Unfortunately, there apparently aren't a lot of medicines on the market that are strong enough to combat anxiety. That's the inspiration behind a new wave of CBD products like those from New York-based cannabis company New Highs."I saw a lot of products that are like 350mg on the market, but what I didn't see was something a bit higher that you needed to take less of," says owner Sarah Remesch, adding that

New Highs tinctures come in both a 700mg bottle and a 2000mg bottle. "I take a few drops from the 700 in the morning and it just balances me. It feels good."

Which goes back to the new conventional wisdom about CBD: It can relax our minds as well as our bodies. Says Ross, "Sure, it's not a cure-all. Maybe it's not for everybody. But because we're all so stressed out and that's causing sickness, people are really responding well to, and benefiting from, CBD."

Waking Up to CBD's Sleeping Powers

There's a very simple reason why the older we get, the more trouble we may have sleeping—and why CBD might help with the problem.

"As we age, we have more issues with sleep, in part because we have more pain conditions as we get older," explains neuroscientist Michele Ross. "So if you're aging and you have arthritis or back pain, that lower back pain is going to wake you up or keep you from falling asleep in the first place."

Beyond pain conditions, there are other factors that can affect sleep patterns in older bodies. Ross notes that "there

are hormonal changes that shorten our sleep cycles. So instead of eight hours, we might be sleeping for six hours, but our body still needs the eight hours. For women especially, it's a problem because in menopause, we have this huge dip in estrogen, which effects our sleep as well."

That's where CBD comes into the picture. Its anti-inflammatory powers can help older people catch added shut-eye by replacing one or more of their prescribed medications (under the guidance of their physician, of course), thus cutting back on

drug interactions that could keep them awake.

This might explain why, in a study conducted by health and wellness website remedy review.com, 61 percent of the seniors who used CBD reported feeling relief from chronic pain—and more than 45 percent said it improved their sleep quality.

"We've had clients who are on 15 medications," says Ross, who also works as a health coach. "Side effects of those medications themselves can also interfere with sleep. So if you can get those patients off one or two medications, it can really make a difference."

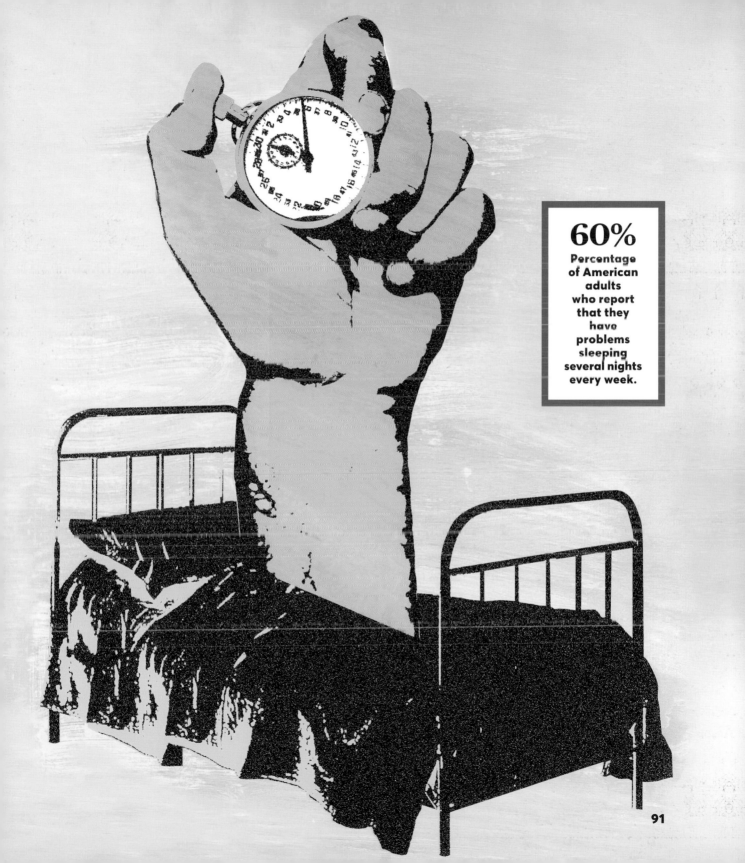

60%
Percentage of American adults who report that they have problems sleeping several nights every week.

SMOKIN' WORKOUTS

Is CBD the new breakfast of champions? Top trainers explain how the plant can improve your regular workout routine.

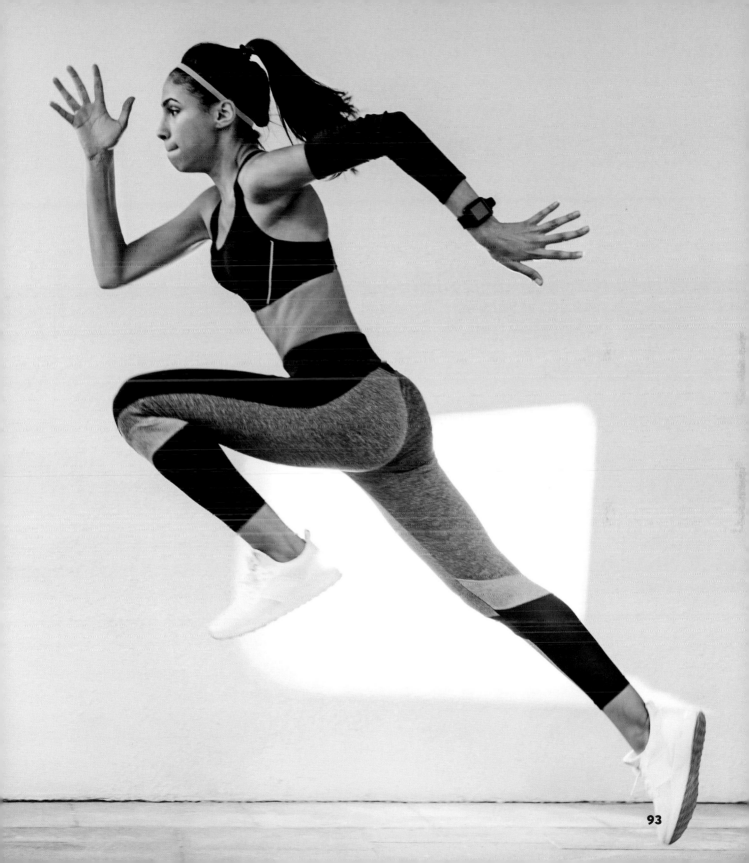

LET'S BE HONEST. When it comes to cannabis and fitness, there is a widely held belief that the closest a regular marijuana user gets to physical activity is channel surfing. Once a run to Taco Bell becomes an official Olympic sport, the stereotype goes, weed consumers will finally have their shot at athletic glory. However, as cannabis' popularity in the U.S. continues to grow, it seems that this plant can be as essential a part of your workout regimen as stretching and wondering if that dude doing the bench press really needs to grunt that loudly.

That's the finding of a research study that was released in April 2019. Conducted by a team of University of Colorado researchers and published in the journal *Frontiers in Public Health*, it involved more than 600 respondents, 81.7 percent of whom said they smoked marijuana before and after their workouts. According to Angela Bryan, senior author of the study and a professor in the school's department of psychology and neuroscience, "There is a stereotype that cannabis use leads people to be lazy and couch-locked and not physically active, but these data suggest that this is not the case."

Other findings: 70 percent of respondents said cannabis enhanced their enjoyment of whatever fitness activity they were doing; 78 percent claimed it boosted their recovery after exercising; and 38 percent believed marijuana use improved their performance. These responses come as no surprise to many in the fitness industry, who have been working some form of THC or hemp-based CBD into their workout routines for years.

"Cannabis has always been popular when it comes to fitness and sports," says Antonio DeRose, co-founder and COO of Green House Healthy, a health and wellness company that promotes cannabis as part of an active lifestyle. "The only difference is, athletes are coming out of the 'green closet' and admitting they consume—because slowly, we are ending the stigma. Professional athletes, weekend warriors and people from all walks of life are finally able to show the world cannabis doesn't make you lazy or stupid. In fact, it benefits our overall health and wellness."

A distance runner and self-described endurance athlete himself, DeRose says he's used cannabis before and after training for races like one that required him and the others on his relay team to run 114.4 miles in under 23 hours. Through his own experiences, he's found that the plant functions as an anti-inflammatory, a pain reliever and a neuroprotectant, while being safer on the body than lab-created drugs like ibuprofen.

"Reducing inflammation quickly without harmful side effects allows for quicker recovery, which can be used to train harder or longer and ultimately improve performance through extra efforts," he explains.

But not everyone is a fan of the psychoactive side of cannabis. Some

4,000

Adults participated in a study that found that those who use pot tend to weigh less than nonusers.

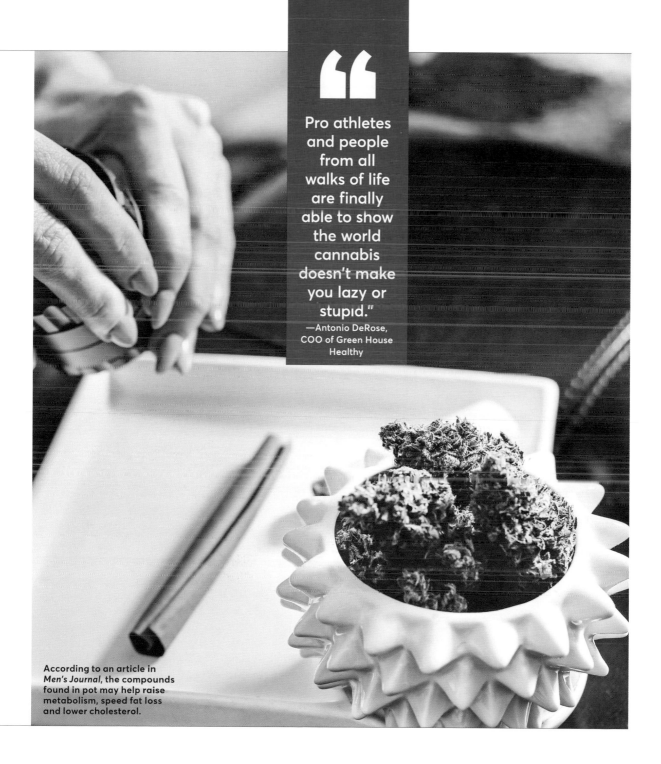

> **Pro athletes and people from all walks of life are finally able to show the world cannabis doesn't make you lazy or stupid."**
>
> —Antonio DeRose, COO of Green House Healthy

According to an article in *Men's Journal*, the compounds found in pot may help raise metabolism, speed fat loss and lower cholesterol.

trainers, like Justin Roethlingshoefer, a strength coach and workout expert whose clients include NHL players, Olympic athletes, celebrities and corporate executives, say users should be cautious with any regimen that incorporates smoking or THC. The former can be unhealthy just on its own, and as for the latter, he says, "There's no reason why you should have a psychoactive ingredient" when you're trying to deal with body aches and pains. Rather, he's a major proponent of using hemp-based CBD-infused oils, creams, rubs and foods.

"The No. 1 reason I talk about CBD is that it can help with certain types of pain," Roethlingshoefer says, noting that this cannabinoid seems to be particularly effective when it comes to aches in joints and muscles. That pain relief can, in turn, leave athletes "feeling a little less run-down. What happens with CBD in oils, balms and tinctures is you have a chemical reaction where it bonds to pain regulators in the body and is able to put you in a more relaxed state. You can be more alert and more focused on what is going on."

As enticing as it might be to try cannabis to help improve your performance, it's also important to first understand what form of the plant may work best for a particular workout. To help find what's ideal for your fitness preference, here's a rundown of various activities and what treatment may make the most sense for each one.

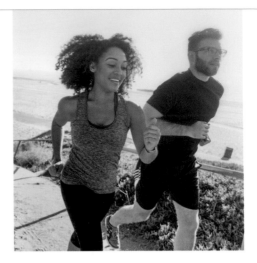

■ Running

According to DeRose, cannabis "can help people get motivated to run, and stay focused during a run.... It also encourages restorative sleep, which helps recovery." Roethlingshoefer adds that because running is an impact sport that puts pressure on your joints and ankles, "you're definitely going to have a little bit more need [for CBD] and see major benefits" thanks to the cannabinoid's ability to reduce inflammation. He and DeRose both suggest using topical creams and rubs, because they can be applied directly to the areas that are sore.

■ Hiking

Because hiking can be as much a mentally soothing activity as a physically demanding one, DeRose believes cannabis is an ideal addition thanks to its "calming and focusing effects that can give us a better appreciation for our surroundings," while also soothing any aching muscles from your jaunt into the wilderness. Stacey Mulvey, founder of Marijuasana, a comprehensive teacher training program for the integration of yoga and cannabis, suggests trying terpene-rich cultivars while going on an intense hike. "Getting into a rhythm is essential with hiking long distances, and cannabis' effect on our cerebellum–the part of our brain responsible for coordinating repetitive movement–can help a hiker drop into one as they are moving," she says.

■ Swimming

This is a nonimpact activity, so there's less need to consume any form of CBD or THC to help with joint inflammation. However, according to DeRose, cannabis (not necessarily just topical) can be beneficial for focus and recovery. "Swimming is a taxing sport on the lungs and some of the major muscles in our bodies," he explains. "We can help calm down our nervous system after an intense swim by incorporating cannabis, which can allow for quicker recovery."

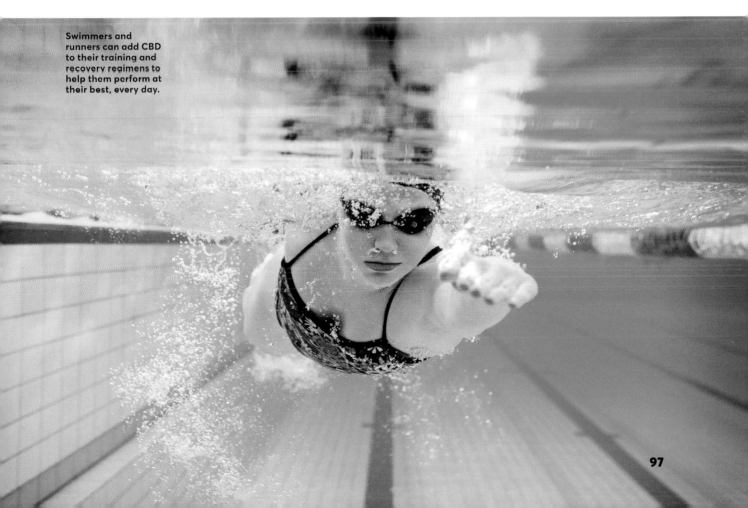

Swimmers and runners can add CBD to their training and recovery regimens to help them perform at their best, every day.

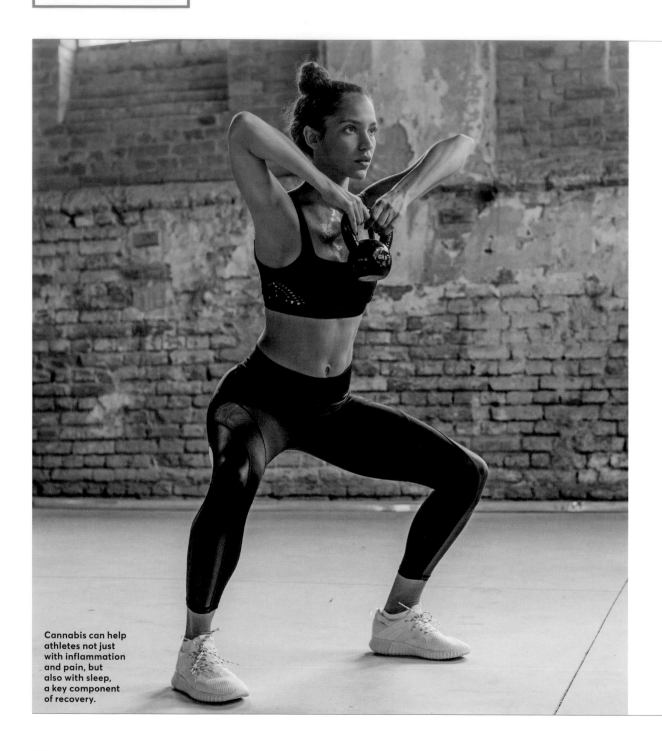

Cannabis can help athletes not just with inflammation and pain, but also with sleep, a key component of recovery.

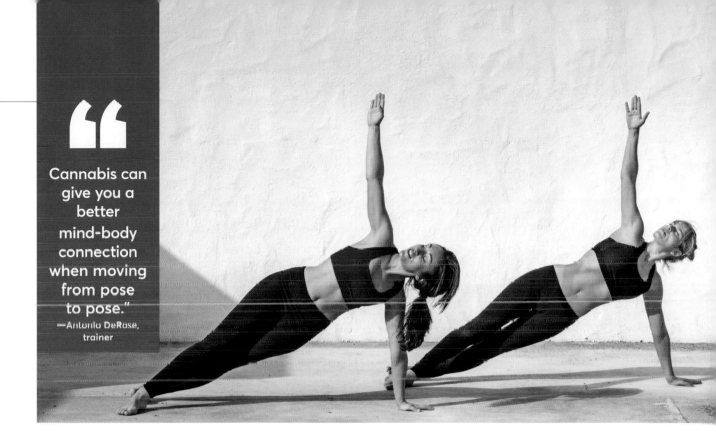

> " Cannabis can give you a better mind-body connection when moving from pose to pose."
> —Antonio DeRose, trainer

■ Weightlifting

Hemp-based CBD can be particularly useful here because weightlifting is likely to lead to things like "isolated range of motion soreness," according to Roethlingshoefer. "Say you have a bench-press day...you might feel soreness in your triceps, chest and shoulders." Creams and lotions can be applied to those areas pre- and post-workout, targeting your upper body for maximum performance recovery. That's a better choice than ingesting a tincture or oil, which provides more of a full-body effect. He also suggests applying some first thing in the morning, particularly on the bottoms of your feet because of sensory neurons that exist there ("It can really change how you feel throughout the day").

However, he cautions not to do this every day because "you don't want to become dependent on them."

■ Yoga

The connection between yoga and marijuana is, not surprisingly, a pretty natural one given the holistic aura associated with both. "Cannabis can help you center yourself to focus on your breathing and give you a better mind-body connection when moving from pose to pose," says DeRose. "This can make yoga more enjoyable, and even more rewarding as a natural healing practice."

That principle cuts right to the core of what Mulvey's Marijuasana is all about, and why a bit of THC in particular might

Some athletes believe that cannabis can improve focus during workouts.

make yoga a more complete experience. "The body responds no differently to incorporating cannabis with the physical practice of yoga than it does to other physical activities," she adds. "However, the inner practice of yoga, which has been described as 'taming the strands of the mind,' is uniquely impacted by psychoactive cannabinoids. This is because the body's endocannabinoid system (ECS) appears to be involved in shifting our perception of the world on an internal level, and in how we show up in relationship and community. Gaining awareness of ourselves and our experience of life is a cornerstone of yogic philosophy."

■ Aerobics

Aerobics is a high-impact athletic activity, so cannabis could be particularly beneficial because its anti-inflammatory properties let you relax before a class and ease the soreness of your stressed joints afterward. Explains DeRose, "Cannabis can motivate many to get started with any aerobic activity. It can help some people overcome pain that may be stopping them from exercising, and for others it just makes exercise more enjoyable. This can make aerobic activities more fun, which will encourage repeating the process, creating long-term positive lifestyle changes that encourage overall health and wellness."

■ Team Sports
(Basketball, football, softball, etc.)

While most major professional sports leagues still ban any cannabis use, even for medical purposes, DeRose notes that the World Anti-Doping Agency has recognized the benefits of CBD as an anti-inflammatory and neuroprotectant by removing the cannabinoid from its banned substance list. "Our ECS is connected to our brain, organs, tissues, glands and cells—so regulating it with cannabinoids is seeming to be beneficial for health and wellness in general," he explains.

What distinguishes cannabis use for athletes involved in team sports, adds Roethlingshoefer, is the regularity of games for your team—which means developing a routine for your cannabis use. "The biggest thing to remember with the team sports you participate in on a 'weekend warrior' basis is to use some type of CBD daily, whether it's a lotion or oil or something else," he explains. "When you have games, you don't want to be sore. You really want to push CBD as your recovery technique versus when you're training or practicing. That's when you might want to back off a bit so when you do have games, you can call upon it in order to feel fresher." Many competitive athletes also say topical CBDs are key in helping speed recovery after a game.

14% Percentage of U.S. adults (about one in seven) use CBD products, according to a 2019 Gallup Poll.

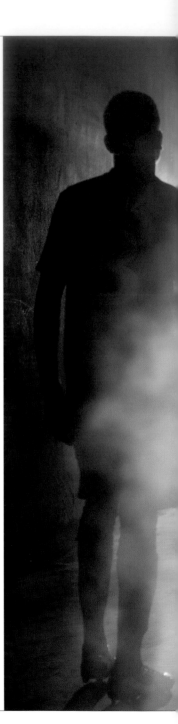

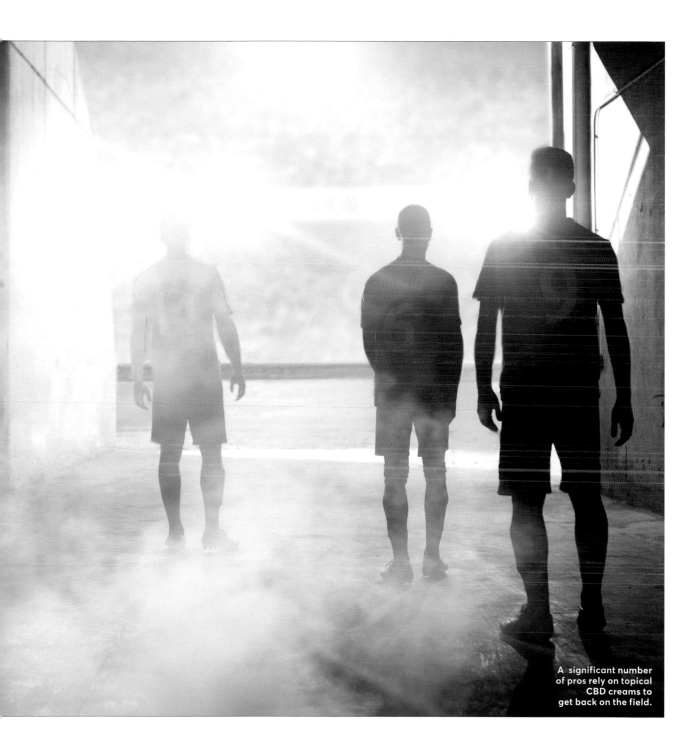

A significant number of pros rely on topical CBD creams to get back on the field.

CUPID'S LITTLE HELPER

CBD supplements and oils just might help you regain your mojo in the bedroom.

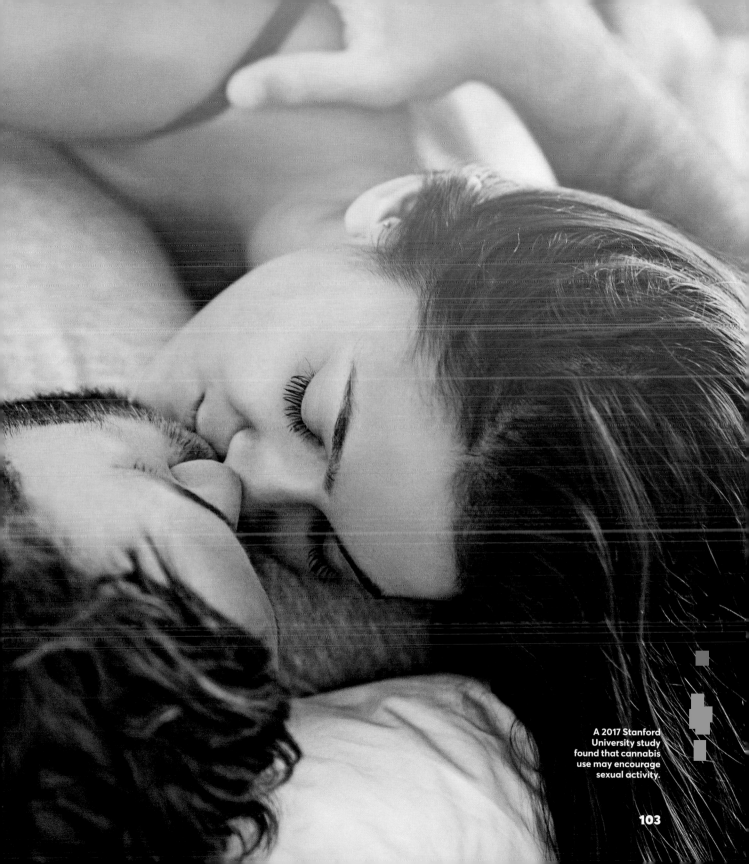

A 2017 Stanford University study found that cannabis use may encourage sexual activity.

FOR CENTURIES, ALCOHOL has been seen as the drug of choice when people want to unwind and get in the mood for sex. But that might not have been the best choice—it lessens inhibitions, but it can actually interfere with the performance of sexual organs. Smoking a joint is not a better option, especially since its high THC content these days can have a deleterious effect on your system thanks to its intoxicating effects. That's why the solution for getting couples in the mood may lie with THC's cannabinoid cousin, CBD. For many, it can be a nonintoxicating way to relax mentally, while also enhancing pleasure and reducing pain.

"There's been an explosion of sex-related CBD products, mostly targeted toward women," says Gretchen Lidicker, author of the book *CBD Oil Everyday Secrets: A Lifestyle Guide to Hemp-Derived Health & Wellness*. "This is mainly due to CBD's calming properties and its ability to combat pain and inflammation, which many women report during and after sex. In addition, a connection has also been established between sexual arousal and the endocannabinoid system, which is the larger system in the body that CBD interacts with."

■ Becoming Cannasexual

Indeed, a 2012 study by the National Institutes of Health showed a significant relationship between endocannabinoid concentrations (your body's natural CBD and THC compounds) and female sexual arousal. Explains Lidicker: "We don't know how taking CBD in supplement form—or infused in massage oil or personal lubricant—might benefit our sex lives directly, but people are reporting positive benefits thus far."

One of those women is Ashley Manta, a self-described "cannasexual" who provides cannabis sex coaching. After six years as a sex educator in Pennsylvania, where she worked with survivors of sexual trauma, she moved to California in 2013 and focused her attention on the pleasure-empowerment side of sexuality.

"I experienced medical cannabis for the first time, and that was a complete game-changer," she says, adding that as a survivor of sexual trauma, it also helped her to experiment not only with CBD but with a THC-infused oil that allowed her to experience pain-free lovemaking "for the first time in well over a decade." Manta had assumed that "[pain] was kind of a fact of my existence" when it came to intimacy, but "an infused product made a huge difference."

■ Buyer, Beware!

As with other CBD products, consumers need to do their research, Manta says, since the marketplace is filled with questionable products thanks to a lack of quality-control standards or regulations.

"There's a lot of snake oil on the market, so it's really important for consumers to do the research and not buy from multilevel marketing organizations that are telling you it's going to cure everything

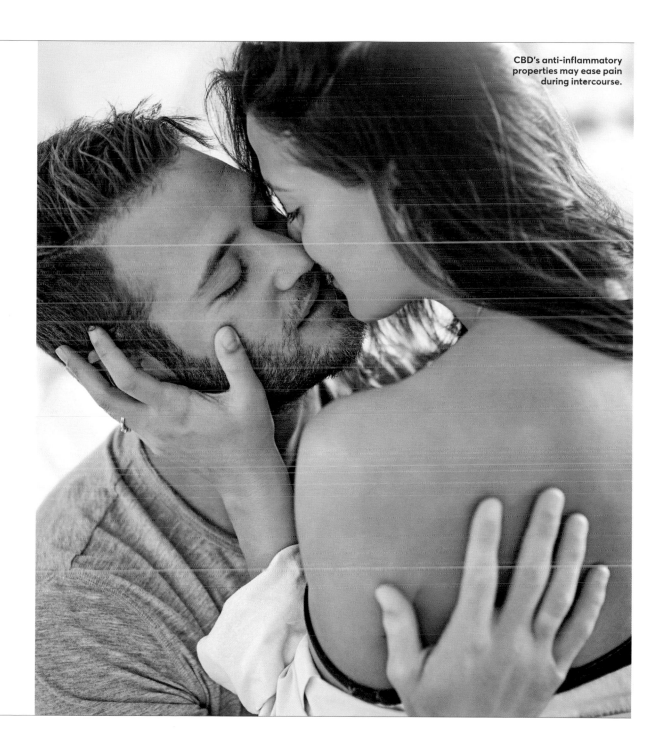

CBD's anti-inflammatory properties may ease pain during intercourse.

from cancer to HIV in three days," she says. "It's important for consumers to be clear on the source, and buy from reputable companies that actually have data to back up their claim."

It's also important to know whether you are purchasing full-spectrum CBD or a CBD isolate. Studies by a leading cannabis research firm, Tikun Olam, have shown CBD-rich products with some THC, along with other plant compounds, work better than just isolates or pure CBD. In theory, any CBD can be beneficial for women's sex lives, considering that their reproductive tracts have hundreds of cannabinoid receptors. That's why applying a topical can allow cannabinoids to get into the tissue and nerve endings, easing pain and increasing pleasure.

■ Kindness, Plus Cannabis

Of course, some old-fashioned thoughtfulness goes a long way, along with an oil or other products. Manta recommends the partner who is less stressed from work and life light candles in the bathroom and draw the other a bath with a CBD bath bomb. While that person is soaking, his or her partner can be tidying up the bedroom and putting on music.

"Perhaps a partner also gives a massage with a CBD oil before commencing in sexy fun times," she says. "That sets yourself up for success in ways [more than] just saying, 'Hey, want to have sex now?'" In other words, you can think of CBD products as just another arrow in Cupid's quiver.

36%
Percentage of U.S. women who have used cannabis in the past six months and say it improved their sex experiences.

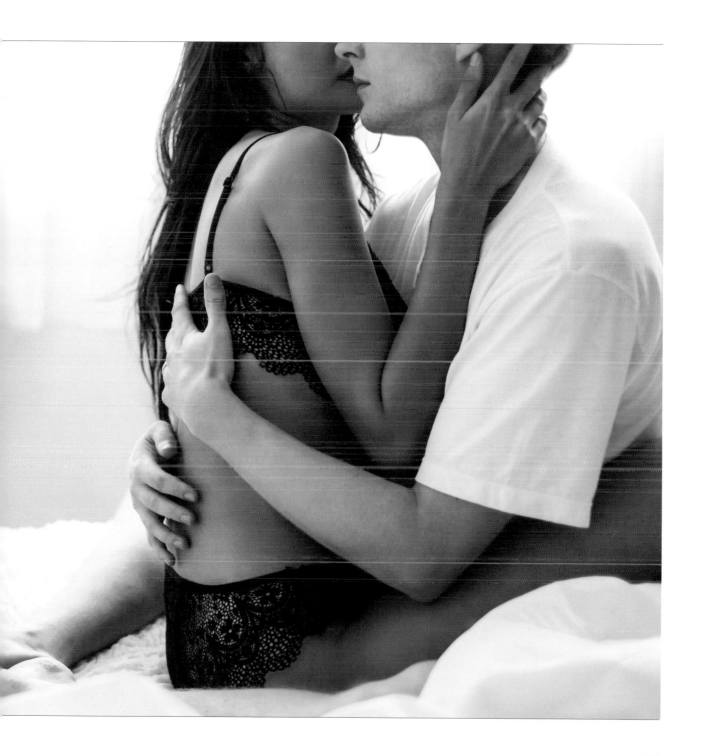

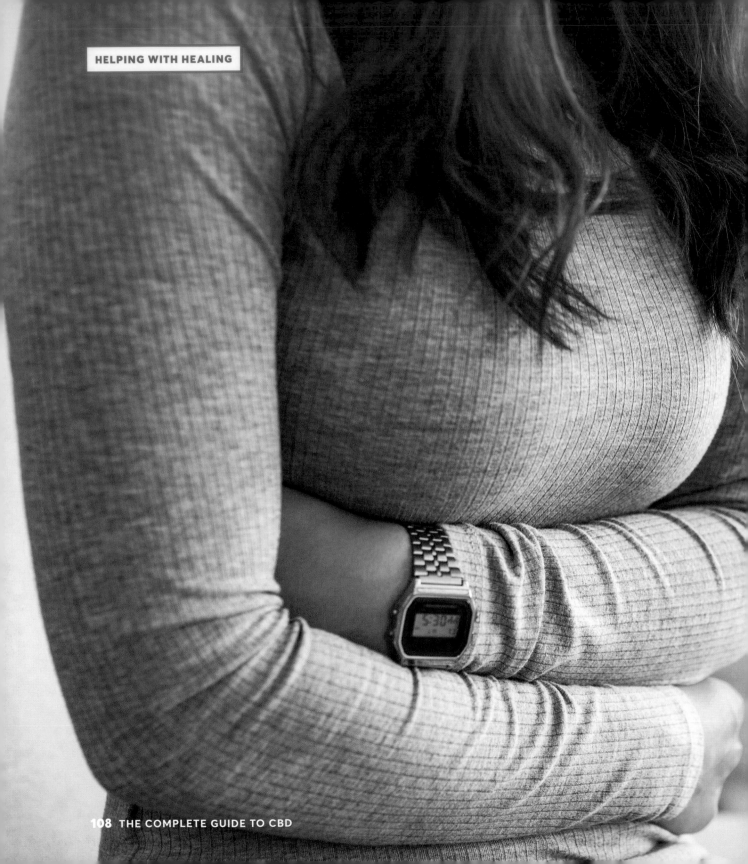

MONTHLY PAIN MANAGEMENT

Is cannabis the smarter way to cope with menstrual discomfort?

THERE IS A WEALTH OF anecdotal evidence that cannabis can help with menstrual pain, and it's been used for that purpose for thousands of years. "There is, however, a lack of placebo-controlled trials to show statistical benefit," says gynecologist Felice Gersh, MD, director of the Integrative Medical Group of Irvine, California, and author of *PCOS SOS: A Gynecologist's Lifeline To Naturally Restore Your Rhythms, Hormones, and Happiness*. "Although lacking definitive proof, there is scientific data to support the mechanism of benefit. Cannabis can definitely reduce pain and inflammation."

Gersh reveals that many of her patients who use hemp-based cannabis to treat painful periods see excellent results. "Highly respected researchers are only just beginning to explore this huge subject," the doctor says. She recommends full-spectrum hemp oil, not an isolate of CBD. "That way, you get the entourage effect," she explains. Gersh is a fan of vaginal suppositories (see sidebar) and products with extra terpenes to control pain.

■ No More Pills

Emily Heinisch, a catering coordinator in Topanga, California, is a regular cannabis user. She describes her monthly cycle as "pretty standard." But over this past year she has experienced menstrual pain within the first 48 hours of getting her period. "I usually wake up in the middle of the night to find that I started my period. That's when the pain is the worst, which makes it difficult to fall back asleep. The next day comes with waves of pain throughout the day. Then the pain usually stops after 48 hours."

Since her teenage years, Heinisch's go-to remedy has been ibuprofen to control bloating and pain, taking about six pills a day. However, as the pain worsened, the nonsteroidal anti-inflammatory just wasn't doing the trick anymore. "So I switched to cannabis. Smoking indica flowers and [ingesting] CBD are a more effective option for me than taking six pills a day to treat the pain," she explains. "I feel the pain-relieving effects much faster by smoking a joint than by ingesting cannabis. Before going to bed or during the middle of the night, I roll an indica flower, because the calming effects help me sleep and relieve pain. And I smoke CBD because it helps with inflammation and bloating during the day."

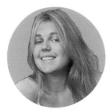

Emily Heinisch

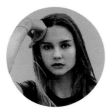

Kirsten Elizabeth

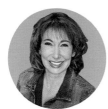

Felice Gersh, MD

Femcare

A London-based start-up, Daye wants to change the rhetoric around periods and women's health. Founded by Valentina Milanova, the company's first product is a CBD-infused tampon. Since there are a lot of cannabinoid receptors in the vagina, it's an easy way to access the plant's pain-relieving benefits. CBD oil also creates a protective sleeve over the tampon; this helps prevent fiber loss, decreasing the risk of bacterial vaginal infection or toxic shock syndrome (TSS). The tampons are created using organic and sustainably sourced cotton, and Daye does not use any plastic in its applicator or packaging. yourdaye.com

■ Finally, Relief

Kirsten Elizabeth is a 21-year-old psychology undergraduate student at UCLA, living in Westwood, California. She's not a regular cannabis user and has a period every six weeks. By the second day she experiences cramping that's similar to a gassy, indigestion feeling, accompanied by nausea. The unpleasant sensation comes and goes for the following three days, in a one-hour-on, one-hour-off pattern.

She doesn't like taking pills regularly, and as a result Elizabeth hadn't treated her menstrual pain in the past; she just suffered. It was only in the past few months that a friend of hers recommended suppositories. Elizabeth immediately felt better, and regretted all the years she'd suffered unnecessarily. It was only after using suppositories for the first time that she had the following realization: The tiredness that accompanied her period wasn't really from the menstruation, but rather from tolerating the pain without any aid.

"The suppositories are incredibly easy to use, and relief comes so fast—and so fully—that I was a little mad at myself for not having figured this out before," she says. "Argh," she playfully wails while throwing her hands up. "Why did I put up with this pain when I didn't have to? At least now, going forward, I know what to do. This year is a big one for me in college and it's good to know I'll be better equipped to focus on my work."

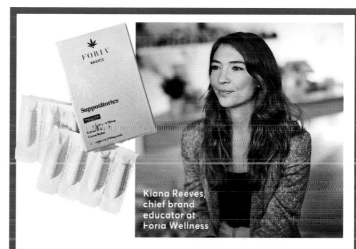

Kiana Reeves, chief brand educator at Foria Wellness

Thinking About Suppositories?

Foria Wellness' Basics Suppositories are formulated for relief during your menstrual period, or for local muscular relaxation and inflammation relief, and can be used vaginally or rectally. Each delivers cannabinoids directly to the muscle and vascular tissues of the upper vagina and uterus.

Foria Pleasure's Relief vaginal suppositories blend THC and CBD and also deliver cannabinoids to the part of the body that needs it most. Kiana Reeves, chief brand educator at Foria Wellness, says women use them from the onset of their cycle, when they're experiencing menstrual cramps, all the way through perimenopause. "We have had customers also use them during pregnancy loss, abortion and postpartum healing."

Suppositories aren't the most common delivery system for medicine in the United States. That's why Foria offers resources to educate the public on the fact that they can be a superior delivery system for certain types of pain management, depending on what part of the body is affected and the type of pain being experienced.

Reeves herself uses suppositories and says, "Typically, day two of my period is the most intense, and I keep a pack of these on hand in my purse and at home so that I am always prepared."

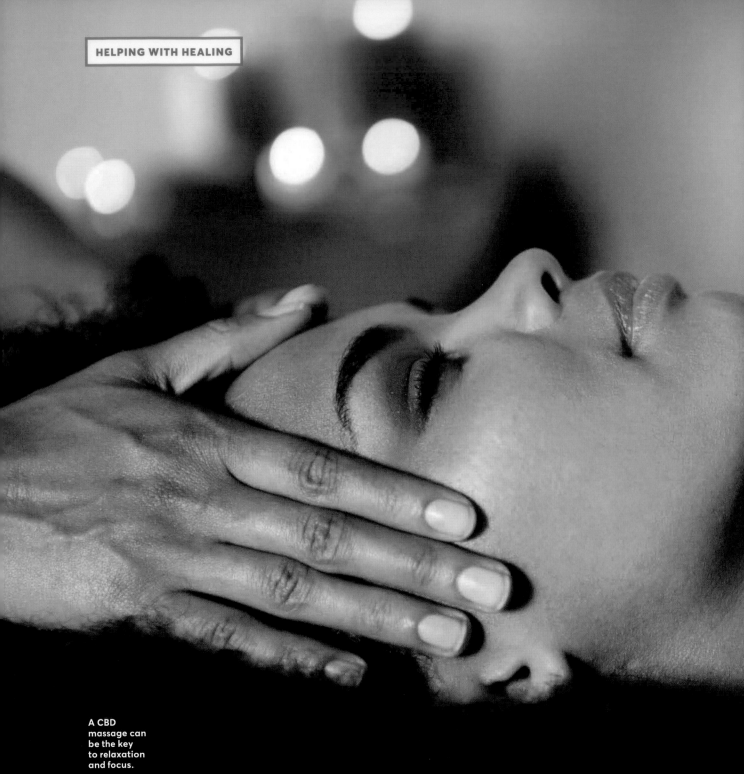

A CBD
massage can
be the key
to relaxation
and focus.

THE HOLY GRAIL OF CBD TREATMENTS

Taking massages to the next level.

AS A WOMAN LIVING WITH multiple sclerosis (an autoimmune condition in which a body's immune cells attack the nervous system), I am always looking for ways to supplement traditional Western medicines to get my errant immune cells to stop wreaking havoc on my body. I've been on a personal search for naturally effective alternative therapies for quite some time (15 years to be exact). In the process, I've been very interested in the rise of cannabinoids–CBD, in particular.

Studies are popping up all over the place, confirming that cannabinoids have a therapeutic effect, both on the symptoms and the underlying neurological damage caused by MS. While my symptoms are relatively mild (numbness and tingling in my hands and feet, low energy levels and a general brain fog that comes and goes)–nothing severe enough for hospitalization or steroids–they're enough to put a damper on my everyday life. And so I dove into the fray to search for ways in which cannabis extracts might help convince my immune system to stop attacking my nerves.

■ Self-research

When I first started looking into it, the cannabis-extract scene was very under-the-radar. Today it seems like you can't turn a corner without running into a CBD latte or a CBD moisturizer. I've tried them all, with varying levels of success; but when I noticed the CBD-massage "Wellness Experience" option at the recently opened Onda Beauty spa in Sag Harbor, New York, I couldn't get there fast enough. And for good reason: This massage was like the holy grail of CBD treatments. It lasted 60 minutes and featured a full-spectrum, 2100mg organic CBD oil (locally produced by a farmer right down the road), which was first worked into my back to maximize absorption and then used in combination with other essential oils and salves.

■ What Happened?

When I emerged, I felt like I had been bathed in fairy dust. Not only were my back and shoulders free of knots, but my hands were less tingly and I was energized and ready to go.

Debra Townes, my therapist, describes our overtaxed bodies as an orchestra, with all the instruments frenetically playing their own tune, out of sync with everyone else. "CBD comes in like a conductor, taps on the stand, and gets everyone to listen and to make music as a unified whole," she explains. "It's not a drug that forces things to be done a certain way. It's a supplement that helps all the systems work in harmony, so we can really address the issues in the tissues. It allows me to go deep, without worrying about causing the muscles too much distress."

Less friction, less stress. Less stress, more energy and clarity. More energy and clarity, better...everything.

Just think of what the world would be like if we were all operating at this level all the time.

–Brooke Williams

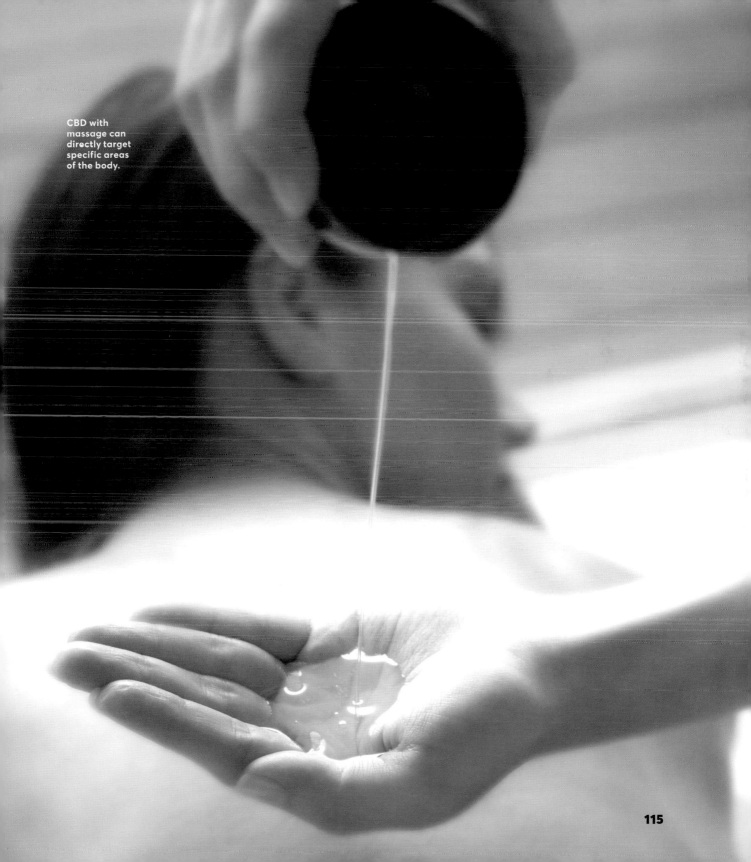

CBD with massage can directly target specific areas of the body.

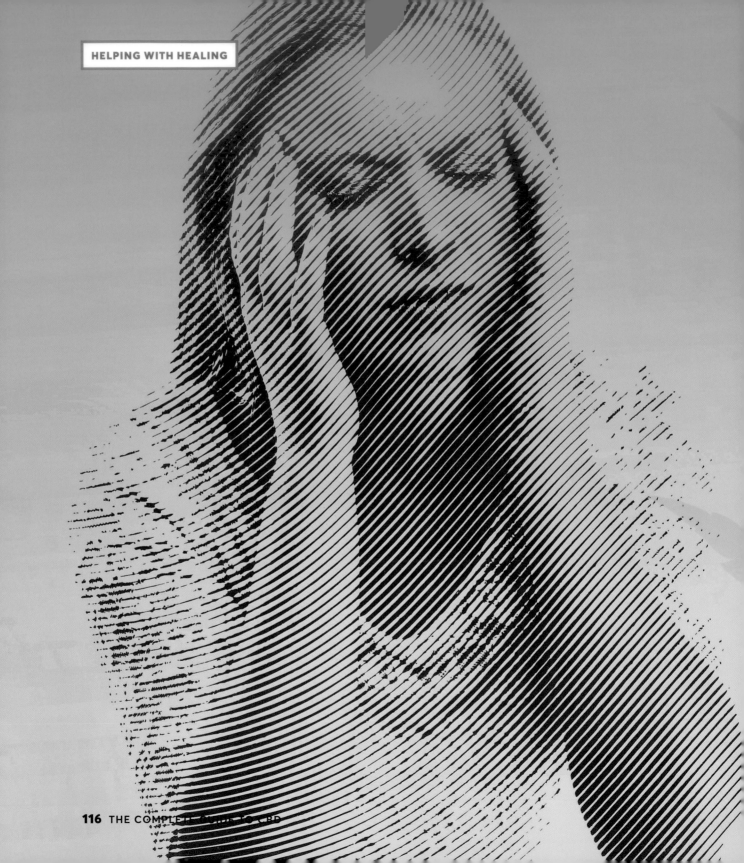

HEAD CASES

Migraine sufferers have started turning to CBD oil to find some pain relief.

IF YOU HAPPEN TO BE ONE of the 38 million Americans suffering from migraines, you know how the experience is to a normal headache what the sniffles are to pneumonia. Migraines arrive with a boatload of symptoms including head pain, nausea, vomiting and a sensitivity to light and/or sound. They are debilitating to the point where 91 percent of those who experience them can't function properly on the job, or simply miss work altogether.

Migraine sufferers have reported trying everything from traditional painkillers to caffeine to yoga to tinted glasses as a way of relieving the intense agony. However, a new and better treatment may be on the horizon: CBD oil. To learn more about how it might help, we spoke with Emma Chasen, a leading cannabis educator and industry consultant.

■ How CBD Can Help

According to Chasen, the unique chemical properties in CBD oil can work as an anti-inflammatory and analgesic within all of our bodies. "It has the ability to interact with many different receptors, enzymes and signaling molecules within the body. This may be because of CBD's ability to help regulate homeostasis, which means bringing the body into balance," she explains.

■ How You Use It

Any trip to a dispensary or a cannabis company's website reveals the many different ways that CBD oil can be ingested. Among the most popular:

- Drops mixed with food or drink
- Capsules
- Inhaling or vaping
- As a topical application directly on your skin

Chasen believes that inhalation is the most effect method for relief, since that approach gets the CBD into your system faster, and migraine sufferers can't wait an extra minute for the pain to stop. However, she is quick to add that "cannabis medicine is personal and therefore the preferred consumption method will be dependent on each individual's needs. Preferred doses will also be dependent on the individual. However, a good place to start is anywhere between 10mg to 20mg of CBD."

■ How to Take It Safely

Many of the studies that have been done on the use of CBD for chronic pain relief were not specifically for migraines, so the research is far from thorough. There's still no conclusive proof it will work to help reduce or relieve your migraines–only anecdotal evidence from those who swear by it. Despite this, Chasen's advice is that it's at least worth a try because there's very little downside.

"With CBD, there aren't many risks associated with the compound itself," she explains. "The most risk comes from the company from which you get your CBD oil. You first need to ask questions like, 'What are their practices? Do they use plant material grown with pesticides?

Are they testing their product for potency, pesticides, heavy metals, etc.?' This is all important to investigate when sourcing CBD oil."

■ How to Take It Legally

If you've decided to try CBD oil, understanding that there's no guarantee it will offer the relief you seek, it's important to investigate whether or not using it is legal in your state. And mostly, says Chasen, "the short answer is yes, it is!" The 2018 Farm Bill, passed by Congress and signed by President Trump, allows for the production and consumption of hemp-based CBD products nationwide, as long as those products fall under one of the predetermined approved categories outlined by the FDA, including containing less than 0.3 percent THC.

However, "CBD derived from medical marijuana is still only available in states with medical/adult-use marijuana programs and may only be purchased at a licensed dispensary," adds Chasen. Make sure to check with your state's health officials to find out the rules that apply, and consult with your doctor to make sure you're doing it safely.

Science Says...
According to the Migraine Treatment Centers of America, CBD oil appears to be able to improve some migraine symptoms for most people.

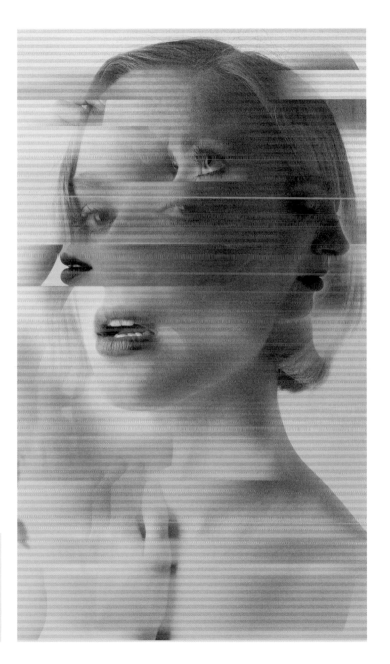

DIY (DOSE IT YOURSELF)

How I learned to stop worrying and try medical marijuana for my back pain.

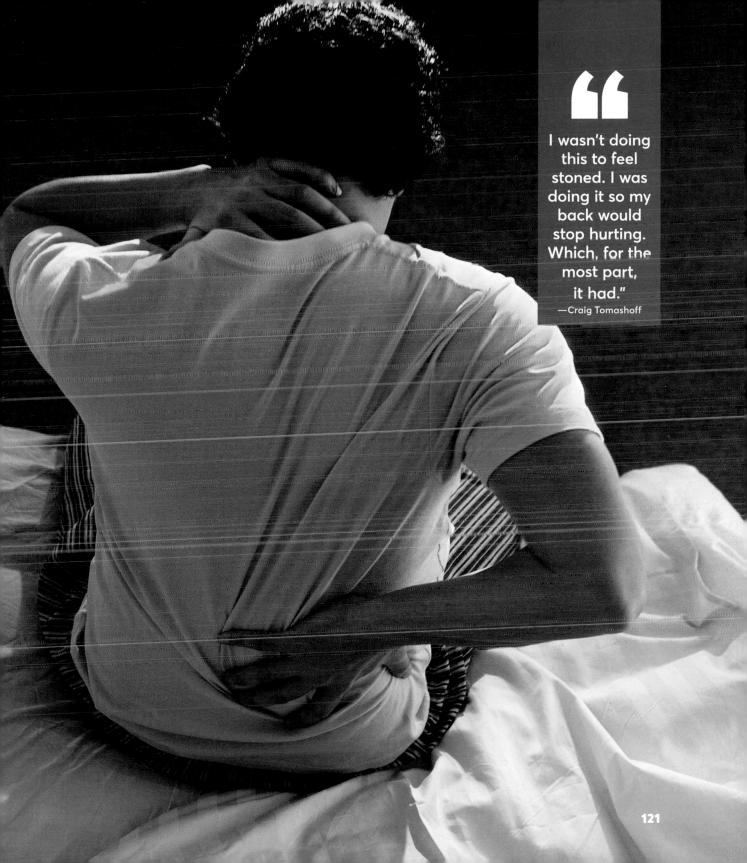

> **"** I wasn't doing this to feel stoned. I was doing it so my back would stop hurting. Which, for the most part, it had."
> —Craig Tomashoff

IT'S SAFE TO SAY, I'M NOT a particularly adventurous person when it comes to drugs. I've smoked marijuana three times in my entire life (and inhaled only once). When my friends in college would light up, I'd suddenly remember an important meeting I had to get up early for. And I don't think I've ever watched two minutes of a Cheech & Chong movie.

Growing up, I'd seen the antidrug PSAs. I'd read the news. I saw footage from Woodstock. In my mind, taking a single hit off a lone joint would leave me trying to take my pants off over my head while hijacking a truck filled with Twinkies. Pot was the devil's plant. Therefore, those who used it were evil as well. Even as public opinion shifted and marijuana–at least the medical version–became socially acceptable, I've resisted trying it, courtesy of my irrational fear. Then I heard from my 80-something mom, who said she'd started using CBD oil for her arthritis. Which she was doing after my brother had started using it for his chronic back pain.

Suddenly, I had no excuse. If the ultraconservative family that taught me drug use was wrong now saw cannabis as an acceptable treatment, I probably should too. And I could use the help. I'd had some major sciatica issues for years now, probably the curse of making a living by sitting at a computer for hours every day. My back had become so painful that when walking my dog, I often had to stop to lie on the ground and do yoga stretches just to make it back home.

■ Fighting the Fear

Surgery and drugs were certainly an option, but frankly, they scared me as much as the sight of a bong. Via a fellow writer's recommendation, I contacted a Colorado company, Infinite CBD (infinite cbd.com). The marketing director, Ali Munk, explained that Infinite had a wide range of hemp-derived CBD products for beginners like me. She reassured me that the products didn't require me getting a medical card and wouldn't provide that Twinkie-munching high I was worried about. Within a week, I received a goody box filled with CBD gummies, drops, oils and lotions, plus a vaping pen.

I set all this out on my desk and then... stared at it for two weeks, still worried that using any of it would leave me couch-bound and craving Cheetos and Grateful Dead music. My kids were tremendously amused that their non-drug-user dad had this little "stash," mocking me for how nervous I got just talking about it. Which was the incentive I needed to finally give in and try CBD.

Bearing in mind Munk's advice that dosing is a tricky thing and everyone should start slow in order to find what works for them, I boldly ate one 25mg gummy. And instantly spit it out. Perhaps it was just my fear manifesting as the taste of mowed grass, but my superior gag reflex took charge. After waiting a few minutes (and feeling a sense of failure), I tried again. This time, the gummy stayed down. I'd been warned it'd take up to 90 minutes to feel any relief. Two hours later, though, my back was still throbbing.

Determined to try again, the next night, I tried one-and-a-half gummies. And 90 minutes in, I still felt nothing. This at first left me discouraged, until I realized...feeling nothing is the point! I wasn't doing this to feel stoned. I was doing it so my back would stop hurting. Which, for the most part, it had. There was still a dull ache but nothing as intense at it sometimes gets. Perhaps it was a fluke, but this was enough to get me to try again the next night.

This time I went for Infinite's Pineapple Express Isolate Dropper. Munk had suggested trying eight to 10 drops under my tongue, to help relax me and curb my back inflammation. Sadly, about three drops in, I mistakenly swallowed everything instead of letting it sit. It tasted like a glass of liquefied pine needles—so, like the first round of gummies, I spit everything out. One night later, I tried again and, this time, managed to get my 10 drops in with no problem. Still, I had to resort to Aleve and a heating pad to curb my backache.

I tried a third time the next evening and again wondered why I wasn't feeling different. Then I tried to get up from the couch to get a glass of water and suddenly realized: I didn't really want to move. My back...hell, all of me...felt more relaxed and comfortable. Maybe it was wishful thinking. Or maybe the drops were actually relieving my pain. Either way, I was happy with the result.

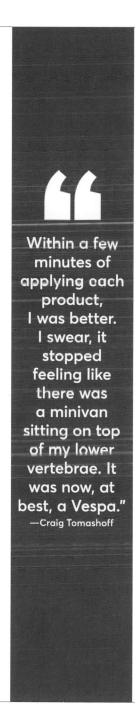

"Within a few minutes of applying each product, I was better. I swear, it stopped feeling like there was a minivan sitting on top of my lower vertebrae. It was now, at best, a Vespa."
—Craig Tomashoff

■ To Vape or Not to Vape

Next up, I began using Infinite's Freezing Point cream and salve, rubbing both liberally into my lower back three or four times a day. This was by far the easiest way to use CBD, because a) there was nothing for me to gag on and b) it literally is no different from rubbing on some Bengay–only without that overpowering smell. Within a few minutes of applying each product, I was better. I swear, it stopped feeling like there was a minivan sitting on top of my lower vertebrae. It was now, at best, a Vespa.

Which brings me to the last item, the vape pen. While eating a gummy or rubbing on a lotion didn't feel like I was doing something immoral, that's exactly how vaping seemed. Still, I'd promised myself I'd try everything, so there was no backing down. I followed Munk's directions, fired the pen up and inhaled as deeply as I could.

■ A Sneaky Sense of Relief

I was expecting to expel that same cloud of vapor we've all seen coming from the tattooed, bearded hipster dude who pulls up next to you at a red light. Instead, though, there was just a pine-flavored burning sensation drifting into my throat. Every expert I'd spoken with about the topic insisted vaping is by far the quickest way to get CBD relief. Fifteen minutes in, though, the only thing that had me feeling worse than the twinge in my back was the lingering cough from inhaling the pen.

I was all set to write about how disappointed I was that vaping didn't affect me at all. Then, once again, I realized relief had snuck up on me. I'd gone an hour without having to stretch out my back or grab the heating pad. I actually felt comfortable, just as I (eventually) had with the gummies, drops and lotions. All I could do was wonder why I'd waited so long for this relief.

Years of anti-pot propaganda had me expecting to become Jeff Bridges in *The Big Lebowski*, so I couldn't accept that that's not what medical marijuana is. It's about getting pain relief, not getting the munchies. Sure, CBD (and maybe a modicum of THC) alone won't cure anyone. It won't help everyone. If you want to heal back pain without opioids and surgery, stretching and exercise are as critical as cannabis-based remedies. Still, ruling out medical marijuana because you can't shake those visions of reefer madness makes no sense.

I may wake up in pain tomorrow, bent over as if I'm about to ring the bell at Notre Dame. Or I may go for a 3-mile dog walk with a smile on my face. Either way, I will be more confident, knowing that I didn't let irrational fear rule my life. I stepped outside my little world, which left me feeling pretty good–spiritually, as well as in my lower back.

–Craig Tomashoff

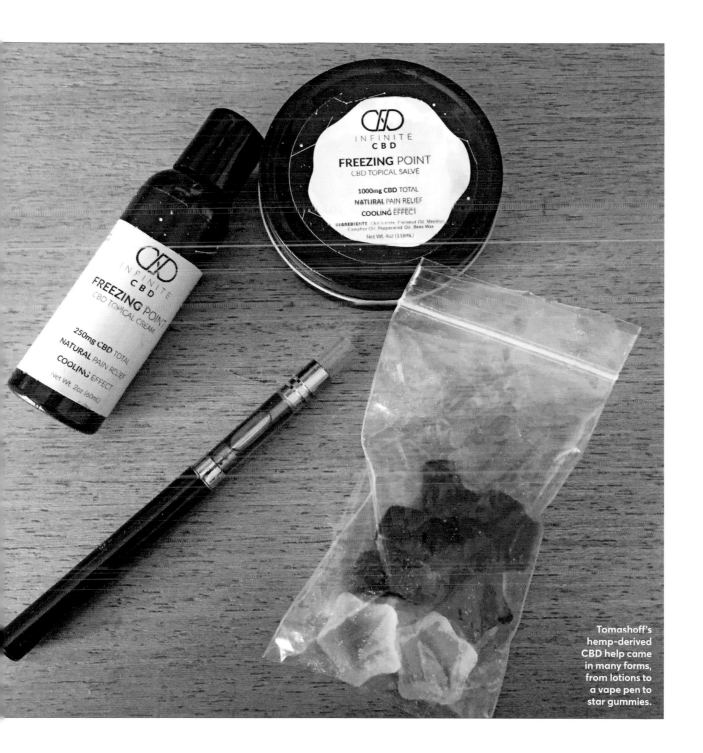

Tomashoff's hemp-derived CBD help came in many forms, from lotions to a vape pen to star gummies.

COPING
WITH
CANCER

The science is still sketchy, but there's plenty of hope that CBD can ease the pain of the disease.

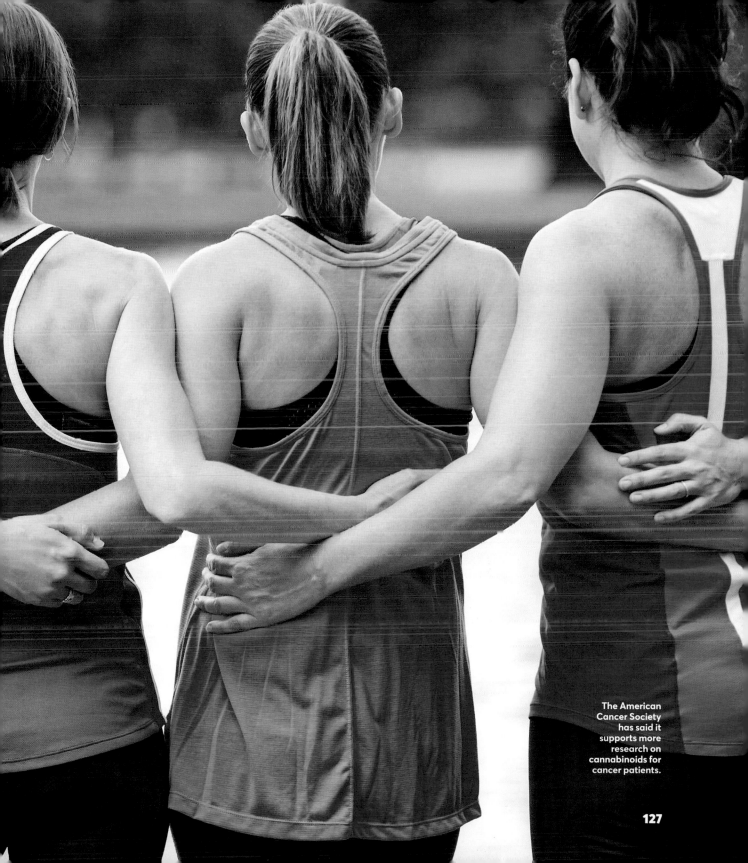

The American Cancer Society has said it supports more research on cannabinoids for cancer patients.

127

WHEN IT COMES TO LEARNING what CBD can do for cancer patients, there are still more questions than there are answers. However, one thing we do know for certain is that many of those who use CBD to treat their cancer, or address the side effects of their disease and treatment, have reported great success. And that anecdotal evidence is enough to give people hope for the future.

"I can see why the public is drawn to a natural alternative that is safe and has a sort of 'people's medicine' kind of vibe to it," says neuroscientist Adie Wilson-Poe, a professor at Washington University in St. Louis who specializes in studying cannabis. "I think as a culture right now there's a backlash against pharmaceuticals and rightfully so—we got ourselves in this huge opioid crisis."

Unfortunately, cannabis' federal classification as a Schedule 1 substance has hindered scientists in the U.S. from researching the full capabilities of the plant. (A lot of what we know has come from research being done in Israel, where there are no significant barriers for scientists who seek to study cannabis.) Because they can't legally conduct significant clinical studies (the kind done on humans), according to Wilson-Poe, there's no way to confirm any claims about CBD's effect on cancer. Nonetheless, there are some preclinical studies (those done on animals and in Petri dishes) that provide some degree of optimism.

"We have a ton of [pre-clinical study] evidence about different components of cannabis that can shrink tumors and interfere with the ability of a tumor to thrive," says Wilson-Poe.

While it's best to remain cautiously hopeful about cannabis' potential to directly impact tumor growth, there are still other already-proven benefits of CBD that may help those suffering from various forms of cancer.

Wilson-Poe notes that THC interacts with our neurotransmitters in an almost identical fashion to opioids, so it provides great pain relief. Meanwhile, CBD interacts with our bodies more like ibuprofen (Advil), so it can work as a powerful anti-inflammatory.

"There's plenty of evidence about CBD's ability to interfere with the body's inflammatory processes," says Wilson-Poe. "So I would say for a cancer patient, that might be helpful with the often extreme amount of pain that typically isn't happening on the surface of the body. It's a visceral pain, a widespread pain and a profound pain. All of CBD's ability to relieve pain is coming from an anti-inflammatory standpoint."

Despite this, though, she cautions that anyone taking prescribed pain medications should be aware of how CBD might interact with those drugs. "If someone is battling cancer, they might be on a number of medications. CBD could either interfere with, or enhance, the ability of that medication to do its job."

CBD can also inhibit certain enzymes in your liver that break up medicine and allow the body to process it. If you interfere with the body's ability to break up medicine, Wilson-Poe explains, "it elevates the amount of medication that's floating around in your bloodstream. That can be a good thing if you're taking a really harsh anti-epileptic drug and you take CBD as well. It means you're inflating the amount of that epilepsy drug in your body, so you could potentially reduce how much of that medication you're taking by supplementing with CBD."

Could this also be the case for chemotherapy drugs? Possibly—but right now scientists just don't know for certain. It will take more time, and potentially the end of cannabis' Schedule 1 designation, before anything can be confirmed. In the meantime, though, Wilson-Poe has good news for anyone looking to supplement their cancer treatment regimen with CBD (after consulting with their physician): "As an add-on therapy to any health regimen, CBD is incredibly safe. With few exceptions, it's not going to interfere with your regular therapy or health."

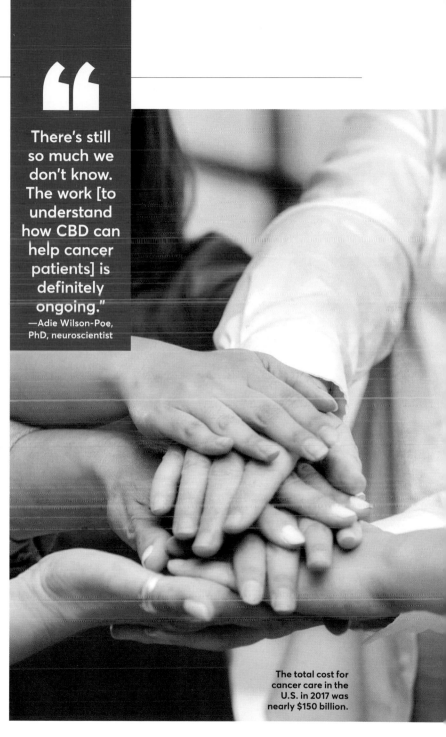

"

There's still so much we don't know. The work [to understand how CBD can help cancer patients] is definitely ongoing."
—Adie Wilson-Poe, PhD, neuroscientist

The total cost for cancer care in the U.S. in 2017 was nearly $150 billion.

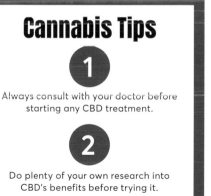

Cannabis Tips

1

Always consult with your doctor before starting any CBD treatment.

2

Do plenty of your own research into CBD's benefits before trying it.

FAREWELL, FEAR FACTOR

CBD is showing a lot of promise when it comes to treating those suffering from PTSD.

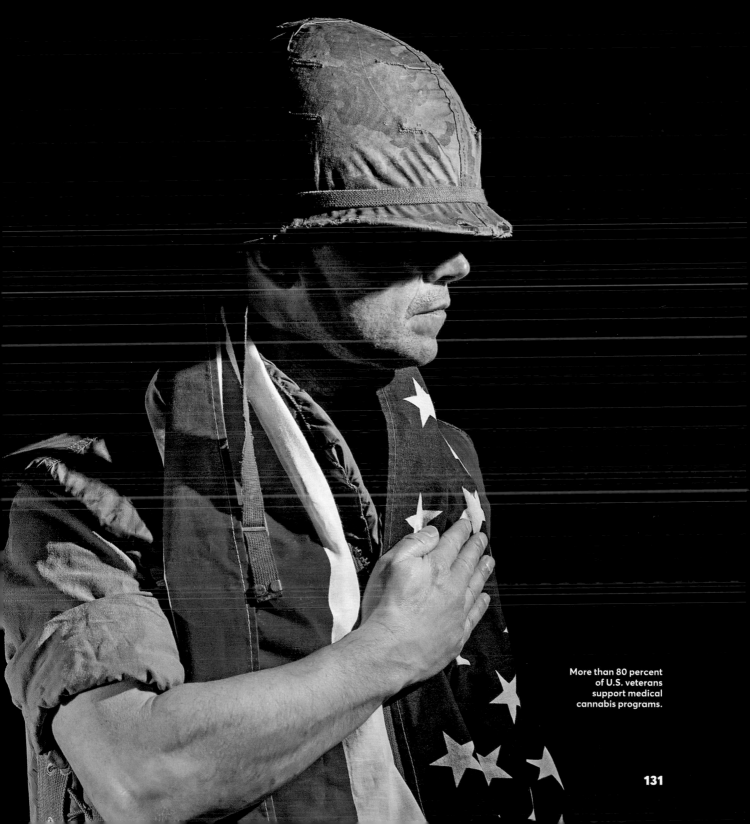

More than 80 percent
of U.S. veterans
support medical
cannabis programs.

BEING INVOLVED IN A CAR crash, assault, military combat or any other violent episode can be damaging enough mentally, as well as physically, for any of us. Now, imagine reliving that incident again and again for months or even years. The experience can leave victims with symptoms ranging from night terrors to insomnia to hypervigilance to incapacitating anxiety. Welcome to the world of post-traumatic stress disorder (PTSD). More than 44 million Americans struggle with it following a disturbing life experience they are unable to cope with. Even the death of a loved one can trigger this chronic psychiatric condition, wreaking havoc not just at work and at home, but in the American economy as well. (The annual cost of PTSD to society is more than $42 billion, often due to misdiagnosis and undertreatment.)

Providing Promise

Unfortunately, most current therapies, such as antidepressants, opiates and anxiolytics (benzodiazepines) aren't effective when it comes to long-term PTSD treatment, and can also have serious side effects. Many patients have said their symptoms got worse with antidepressants or narcotics. Then, along came the discovery of the endocannabinoid system (ECS) and its role in emotional memory processing. This has created hope for PTSD via pharmacological manipulation of the ECS, and that means using CBD, which has a direct effect on that system.

"Out of all the mental health disorders, CBD might show the most promise for PTSD," says Gretchen Lidicker, author of *CBD Oil: Everyday Secrets: A Lifestyle Guide to Hemp-Derived Health and Wellness*. "Cannabinoids like CBD have the potential to both modulate memory processing and reduce anxiety and depression—with virtually no side effects. And considering the fact that one in 10 people will be diagnosed with PTSD, this is a big deal."

Studies by the National Center of Biotechnology Information (NCBI) have suggested PTSD sufferers have lower levels of anandamide, an ECS molecule known to reduce stress and promote well-being, like what people feel after exercise. "As observed in rodents," a 2018 NCBI report noted, "recent studies have confirmed the ability of CBD to alter important aspects of aversive memories in humans and promote significant improvements in the symptomatology of PTSD."

Clearly, more research needs to be done, but the preliminary studies and anecdotal evidence both look very promising, providing hope for people who currently have very little.

"The clinical research just isn't there yet—mostly due to the many barriers to studying CBD on humans in the U.S.—but surveys and patient reports suggest that people who have access to high-CBD cannabis are not only using it—but it's working," says Lidicker. "They report that cannabis was most likely to improve PTSD symptoms and least likely to make them worse, and that [patients] were able to reduce their need for other medications and substances, like alcohol, if they used cannabis."

5%

Percentage of Americans who are suffering from PTSD at any given moment.

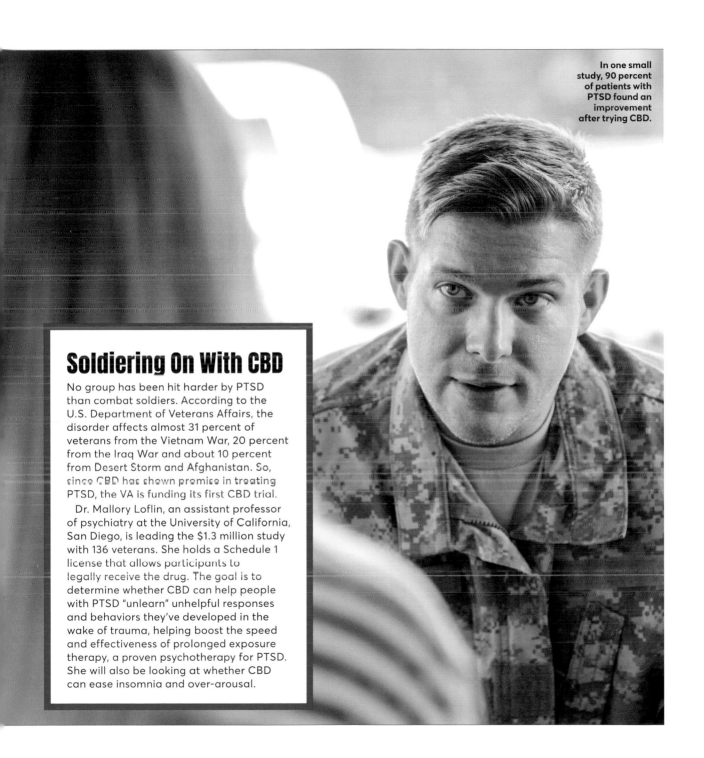

In one small study, 90 percent of patients with PTSD found an improvement after trying CBD.

Soldiering On With CBD

No group has been hit harder by PTSD than combat soldiers. According to the U.S. Department of Veterans Affairs, the disorder affects almost 31 percent of veterans from the Vietnam War, 20 percent from the Iraq War and about 10 percent from Desert Storm and Afghanistan. So, since CBD has shown promise in treating PTSD, the VA is funding its first CBD trial.

Dr. Mallory Loflin, an assistant professor of psychiatry at the University of California, San Diego, is leading the $1.3 million study with 136 veterans. She holds a Schedule 1 license that allows participants to legally receive the drug. The goal is to determine whether CBD can help people with PTSD "unlearn" unhelpful responses and behaviors they've developed in the wake of trauma, helping boost the speed and effectiveness of prolonged exposure therapy, a proven psychotherapy for PTSD. She will also be looking at whether CBD can ease insomnia and over-arousal.

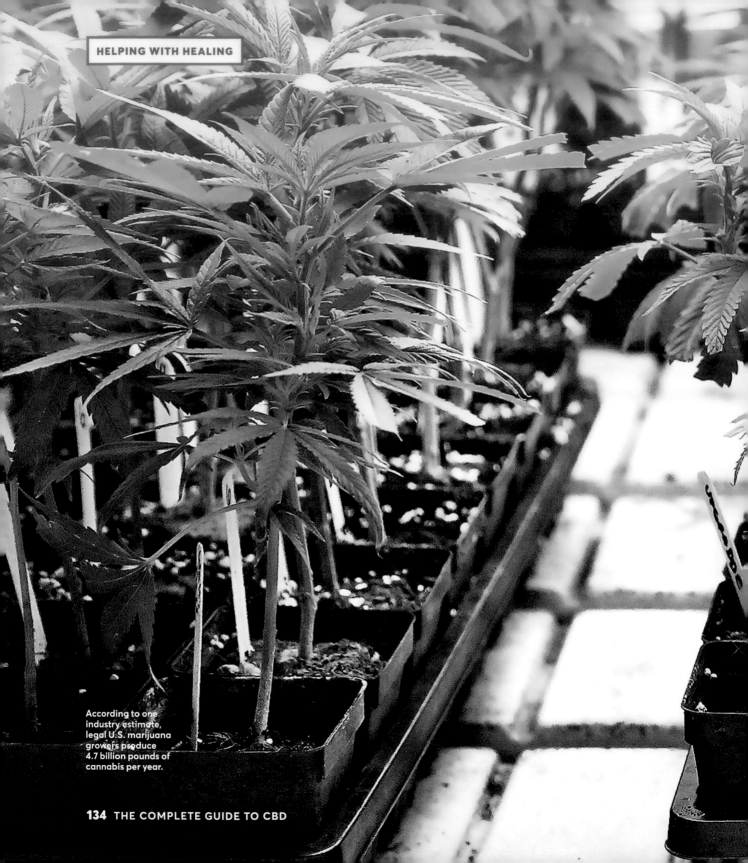

According to one industry estimate, legal U.S. marijuana growers produce 4.7 billion pounds of cannabis per year.

COMING CLEAN

It seems like a savior, but some CBD may be doing you more harm than good.

THERE'S NO DOUBT THAT the world has gone all in on the cannabis craze, including CBD. Polls routinely find that U.S. approval for complete legalization is in the mid-60 percent range, while a March survey from Quinnipiac University discovered that 93 percent of Americans favor legalizing medical marijuana. Meanwhile, worldwide legal cannabis sales topped $12 billion in 2018.

The plant is certainly popular, and the purported positive effects of CBD are one of the major reasons for this surge. However, it turns out that not all cannabis is created equally. Whether it's due to poor growing techniques, negligent cultivation or unnecessary additives, plenty of pot on the market could potentially be bad for you. According to Shira Adler, author of *The ABCs of CBD: The Essential Guide for Parents (And Regular Folks Too)* and founder of the health and wellness company Synergy by Shira Adler, there's the very real possibility that "you can run the gamut from something as simple as not getting the CBD amount you thought you were getting to something much worse. You're getting a product that could have mold, toxins, pesticides, solvent residues.... I know someone who had a bad reaction to a tincture because the CBD was not clean anymore." So what exactly constitutes "clean CBD?"

"Clean CBD means that the cannabis or hemp that the CBD was extracted from wasn't treated with plant-growth regulators (PGRs) or pesticides while the plants were cultivated," says Robert Flannery, who has a PhD in plant biology and is founder of the "clean cannabis" company Dr. Robb Farms.

Unfortunately, the more popular CBD becomes, the greater the likelihood of it being tainted. At least that's the opinion of Brad Bogus, growth and marketing vice president for Confident Cannabis, whose software has created a database analyzing cannabis that's legally available around the world. This means there's a good chance you might not be getting what you're paying for when it comes to CBD.

"The problem is much worse," he explains. "We've seen numerous products offered on Amazon test with little to no CBD potency present, while those same products list 1000mg on the bottle. You can't trust a company that doesn't test its own product or come out straight about what's in it. We've seen how very quickly the vape market developed high-THC products and what kind of toxic additives have been discovered since that [happened]. CBD is probably 10 times that. This will settle down eventually, but you can't trust any company with any product just anywhere."

■ The Risks

Flannery says he's seen people who took ill from bad CBD, like the patient who starting having severe headaches and shortness of breath after vaping a cartridge which turned out to be tainted

The Responsibilities

Because there is still not a lot of stability when it comes to the patchwork of state cannabis regulations, it's incumbent on anyone who is interested in using CBD to look out for themselves. That's why plant biologist Robert Flannery's advice is pretty simple—always purchase your products from a licensed dispensary.

"Buying from the legal market will ensure that your CBD product isn't also coming with plant-growth regulators (PGRs) and pesticides," he explains. "There are regulations in place to ensure that. The system isn't perfect by any means, but buying from a licensed dispensary is the best way to feel confident that your CBD products are clean."

Cannabis software marketer Brad Bogus also suggests taking things one step further, going online to verify a particular brand's credibility because "this is one area you want to invest a little more time in than the usual reading of buyer reviews. Treat it like you would if you were shopping for a laptop or TV." If you want to be extra sure about the quality of your cannabis, Bogus has one more idea that might seem extreme, but usually gets you what you need.

"Contact the company. This may seem brazen, but the cannabis community is proud to back up their product and happy to share information about it," says Bogus. "Companies that are unapproachable or just tight-lipped about their product and testing are not to be trusted. But you can reach just about any company's CEO if you want through their online contact form. Just ask."

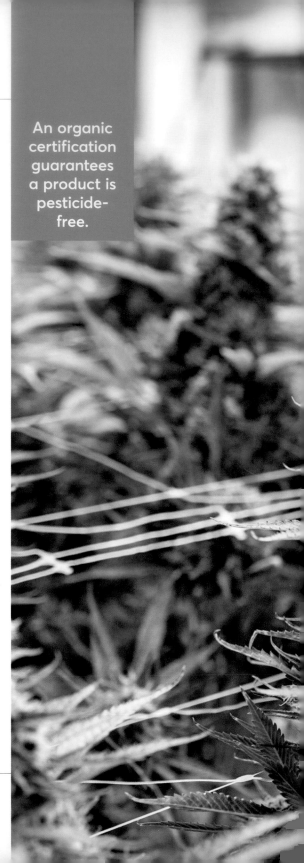

An organic certification guarantees a product is pesticide-free.

with a toxic fungicide that released hydrogen cyanide when heated. However, Bogus does have some good news: The kinds of contaminants that could show up in cannabis medicines are at least not life-threatening. "While you can't trust the cleanliness of anything on the market," he says, "there isn't heavily toxic CBD out there that will poison you or give you cardiac arrest or anything." Still, perhaps the greatest danger from contaminated CBD is that it might scare people from giving the medicine a chance to do what it does.

"Buying bad CBD will absolutely discourage people from using it," Bogus explains. "This is a substance that people are highly curious about but also have a lot of trepidation to try. So when a person who is just barely convinced that they should try this product gets a bad or, more likely, ineffectual product, they'll assume it was all snake oil and confirm those biases."

■ The Regulations

On the plus side, the more states legalize medical cannabis, the more regulations there are out there to ensure you're getting pristine, legal CBD. Nonetheless, there's no federal standard for marijuana-derived CBD since cannabis is still a banned substance. (The 2018 Farm Bill, passed in December, establishes a framework for the federal sales and regulation of hemp-derived CBD, as long as it has less than 0.3 percent THC.)

"We live in a time where cannabis is regulated in places like California, Colorado

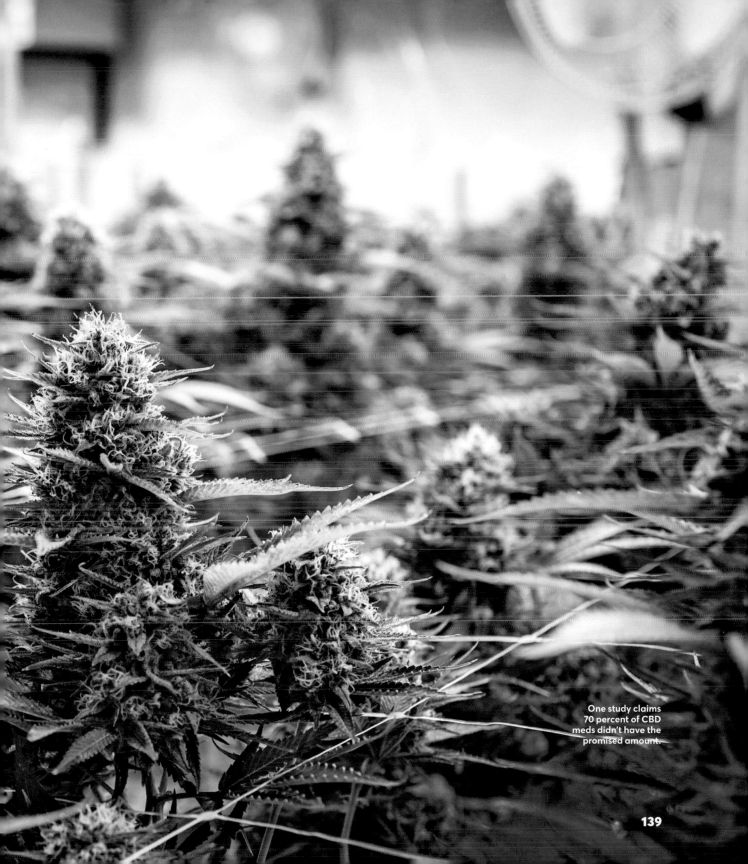

One study claims
70 percent of CBD
meds didn't have the
promised amount.

or any of the other states that have legalized some form of cannabis consumption," says Flannery. "In the regulated markets, it's required for the cannabis to be tested by a third-party laboratory to see whether or not it's clean. The labs also test the product for potency. This is a good indicator of what you can expect when it comes to how much CBD is present in the flower."

If you're buying from a respectable company, adds Bogus, it will link all its products to test results from licensed labs. For instance, "one of my favorite brands, Bluebird Botanicals, has batch-level test results you can find on their website linked right from every bottle. I expect this standard for any good CBD company."

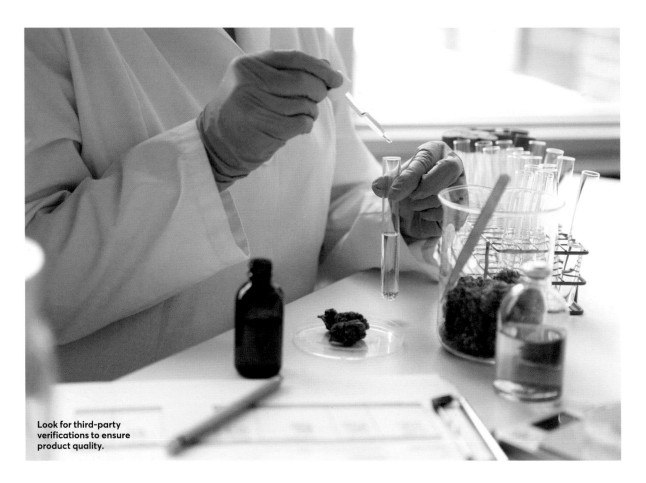

Look for third-party verifications to ensure product quality.

Decoding the Label

While it's important to read the label of any medicine you're going to take, it's even more critical when ingesting something containing CBD since cannabis industry regulations are still (literally) all over the map. To learn what you need to look for before buying your CBD medicine, we asked Shira Adler, CEO of Synergy by Shira Adler, to break down one of her product labels as a way to teach consumers exactly what to look for before they make a cannabis purchase.

TYPE AND STRENGTH
This entry indicates the predominant type of medicine (a tincture, in this case), as well as the total amount of CBD that is contained in the entire bottle.

WHAT IT'S FOR
Companies can't make medical claims with over-the-counter products—so this line should say "supplement."

WHAT YOU GET
This is basic information about the volume of what's inside. If it's missing, that's a reason to avoid purchasing it.

SERVING SIZE
This entry will list the exact amount of CBD that's in each serving, as well as how many servings you'll get in the container.

WHAT'S INSIDE
This is a section that should be read carefully. It has to list everything within the container, so consumers should keep an eye out for ingredients that hinder product quality, such as sweeteners.

QUALITY CONTROL
This Good Manufacturing Product label indicates that the manufacturer is legitimate.

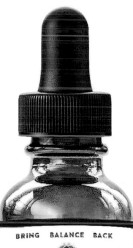

BRING   BALANCE   BACK

SYNERGY
BY SHIRA ADLER

**CBD TINCTURE
1500 MG**

DIETARY SUPPLEMENT

Recommendations: Take half dropper up to twice a day, or additionally as needed for desired effect. Drop between cheek & gum. Absorbs in seconds. Follow with 2-3 spritzes of our signature Aromatherapy Synergy Sprays as part of our complete holistic regimen.
Warning: If pregnant or nursing, consult your health care practitioner before using this or any other CBD product.

 1 FL OZ (30 ML)

Supplement Facts:
Serving Size: 15 Drops
Servings Per Container: 60

Amount Serving:
Cannabidiol (Total CBD): 25 mg

INGREDIENTS:
Organic MCT oil & Organic Full Spectrum Hemp Extract.

OTHER FACTS:
Free of GMO, Gluten, Color, Additives & Preservatives

Distributed By:
Diva Mama, LLC
292 Katonah Ave #412
Katonah, NY 10536
ShiraSynergy.com

© 2019 Diva Mama, LLC

GMP QUALITY PRODUCT

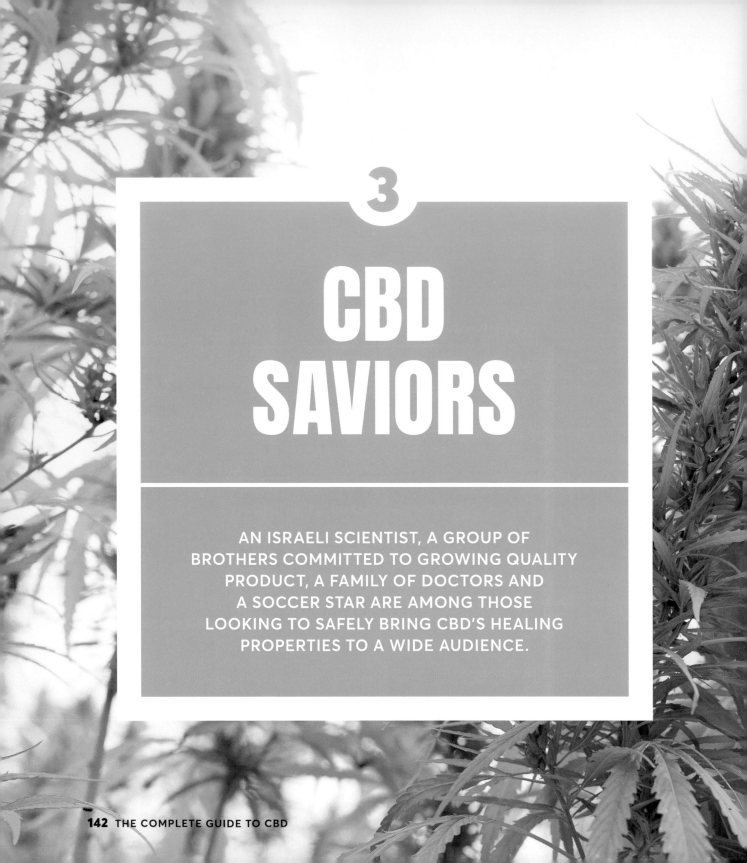

3

CBD SAVIORS

AN ISRAELI SCIENTIST, A GROUP OF BROTHERS COMMITTED TO GROWING QUALITY PRODUCT, A FAMILY OF DOCTORS AND A SOCCER STAR ARE AMONG THOSE LOOKING TO SAFELY BRING CBD'S HEALING PROPERTIES TO A WIDE AUDIENCE.

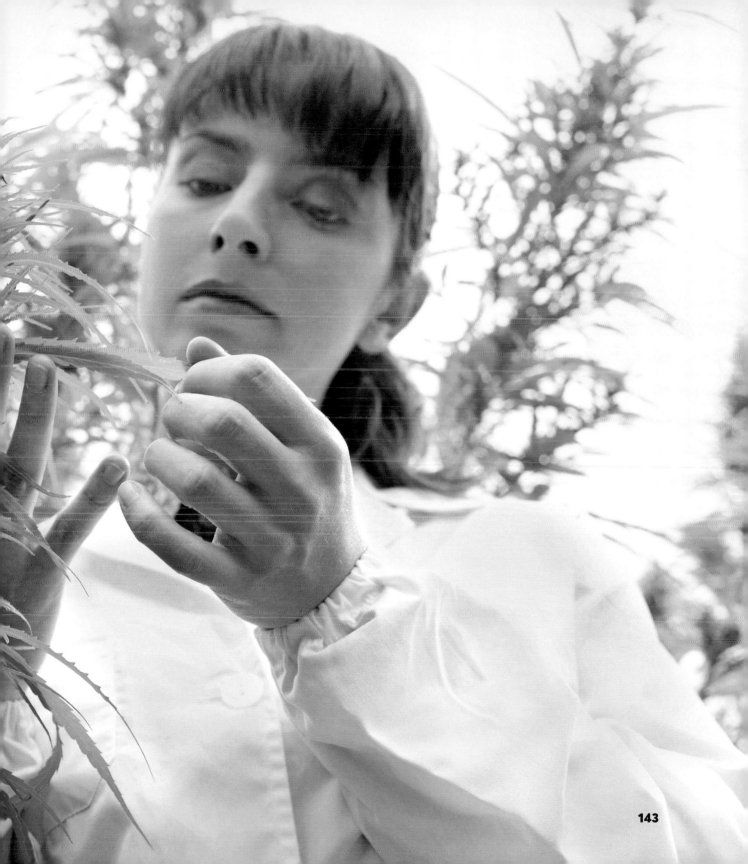

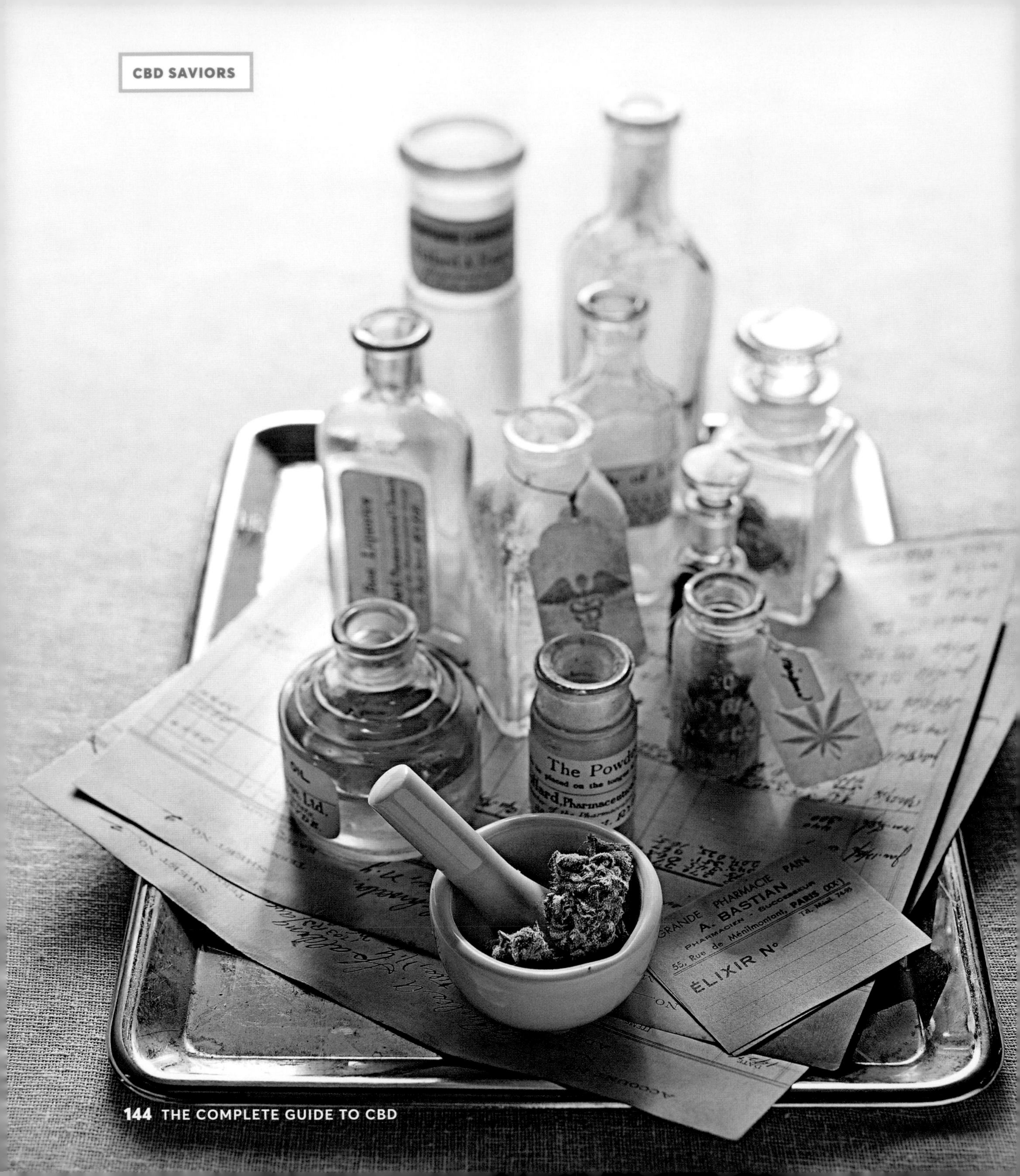
A. BASTIAN
ÉLIXIR N°

IN THE BEGINNING

For years, the cannabis plant was a mystery, until a young
Israeli researcher decided to find out what made it tick.
Almost 60 years later, Raphael Mechoulam's groundbreaking
work is inspiring an exciting medical revolution.

ANCIENT CIVILIZATIONS knew that when ingested, the flower of the cannabis sativa plant eased pain, inflammation, epilepsy and other maladies. Of course, they couldn't help but notice that the plant also had something in it that was mood-altering.

Over the centuries, cannabis and its resin, hashish, became more widely known for the high they induced than for their healing properties. Nation after nation outlawed the "devil weed" in the 1800s and 1900s. As a result, modern scientific researchers simply couldn't obtain samples or funding to study the plant's pharmacology and chemistry. It took a bit of Israeli chutzpah to break the deadlock.

If today the many medical benefits of cannabis are gaining recognition and causing governments to rethink policies, much of the credit goes to Raphael Mechoulam, PhD, an Israeli researcher. In the early 1960s, Mechoulam, then a new member of the chemistry faculty at the Weizmann Institute of Science in Rehovot, a city near Tel Aviv, discovered plenty of old cannabis research that had been conducted in several countries. But the plant's active compounds hadn't

Israel has become a world leader in researching the medical benefits of marijuana.

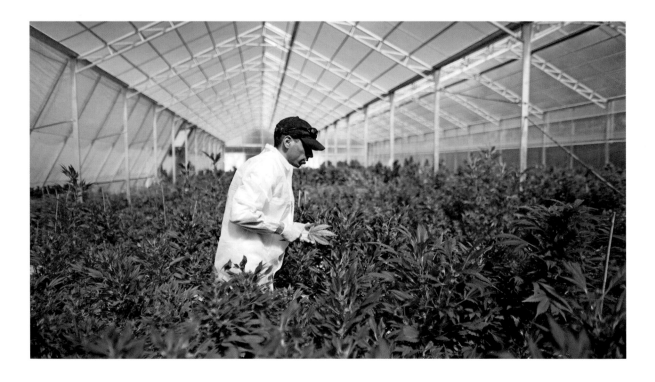

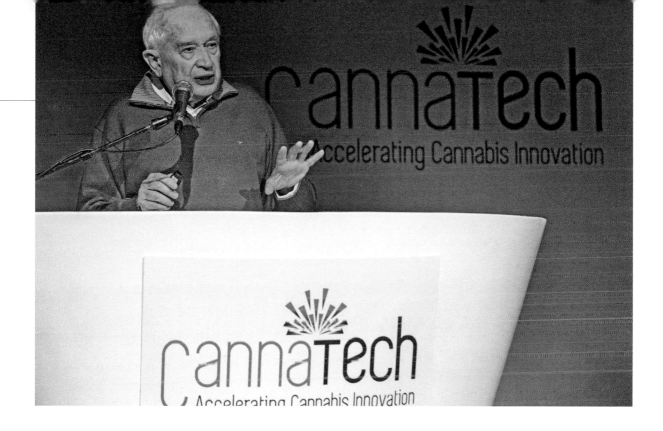

been isolated, synthesized and analyzed in pure form, and studies had screeched to a halt due to the criminalization of pot.

■ Calling the Police

Mechoulam was eager to reopen the field for investigation by using then-new methods such as nuclear magnetic resonance spectrometry. One problem: how to get samples? He asked the institute's administrative director if he knew anyone at police headquarters. Well, yes—as a matter of fact, the director had served in the military with the officer who at the time headed the investigative branch of the Israel National Police. And that's how he ended up on a bus from Tel Aviv with 11 pounds of high-quality Lebanese hashish that had been seized from smugglers.

Mechoulam and his police contact later learned that their arrangement wasn't strictly legal, but they were permitted to continue once Mechoulam apologized and got a proper license from Israel's Health Ministry.

"Working in a small country certainly has its positive aspects," Mechoulam commented. "It couldn't have happened in the United States because the laws were too strict. In Israel, there's a lot of shouting, but at the end you can make it."

Mechoulam and his research partners, Yuval Shvo and Yechiel Gaoni, used their stash to isolate several of the plant's 142 active components, map their structures, synthesize them and make them available for pharmacological and clinical research. Mechoulam coined

Cannabis research pioneer Raphael Mechoulam (above) is a Holocaust survivor.

the term "cannabinoids" to describe these compounds.

The most significant cannabinoids they isolated and mapped, in 1963 and 1964, were cannabidiol (CBD) and tetrahydrocannabinol (THC). CBD is now known as a potent anti-inflammatory and anti-anxiety agent; psychoactive THC turns on the receptors in the body that may alleviate symptoms and help heal numerous conditions. Mechoulam's group reasoned that if the body has cannabinoid receptors, the body must also have biological cannabinoid-like compounds that are endogenous, meaning already inside us.

Sure enough, in the early 1990s, Mechoulam's team identified the enzymes, receptors and cannabinoid-like natural compounds (endocannabinoids) that constitute what they called the endocannabinoid system (ECS) we're all born with. (Fun fact: The female reproductive system contains the most endocannabinoid receptors, second only to the brain.)

It turns out the ECS "is involved in a huge number of functions," said Mechoulam. And theoretically, tinkering with the ECS could have huge therapeutic potential. "The discovery of the ECS, coupled with the upsurge in cannabis use throughout the world, led to a major expansion of research in this field," he added.

■ Cannabis and Autism

Now 89 years old, Mechoulam still works in his lab at the Hadassah Medical School at the Hebrew University of Jerusalem. Surprisingly, much of his funding over the past 50 years has come from the United States National Institute on Drug Abuse, because clinical cannabis research in the U.S. (and other countries) remains limited despite varying degrees of legalization. In contrast, Israeli researchers can not only get a wide range of plant strains from government-certified cannabis growers, but also mine valuable patient data from thousands of prescription medical cannabis users dating back to the early 1990s. Israel has become a global powerhouse in cannabis cultivation, technology and scientific research.

"There are over 120 clinical trials involving cannabis going on in Israel now," says Saul Kaye, founder and CEO of iCAN, an Israeli firm that identifies and accelerates innovative companies in the medical-cannabis space to promote a global cannabis ecosystem,

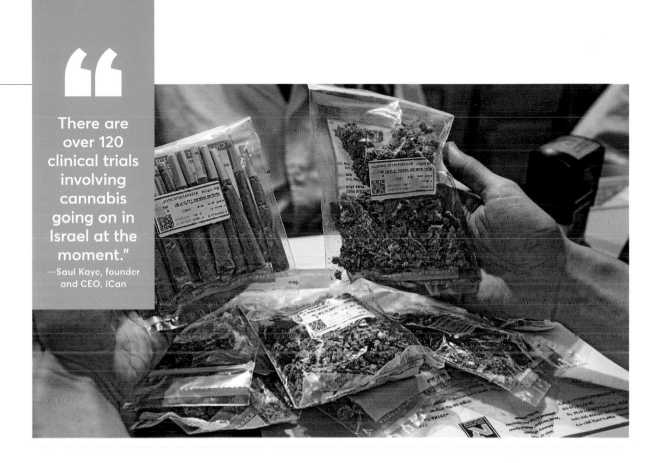

endocannabinoids (from humans) to find effective treatments for a huge variety of ailments, among them: arthritis, asthma, autism, brain trauma, broken bones, cancer, chronic pain, Crohn's disease, type 1 diabetes, endometriosis, epilepsy, fibromyalgia, glaucoma, graft vs. host disease (GVHD), heart disease, insomnia, irritable bowel syndrome, chemotherapy-related nausea, Parkinson's disease, post-traumatic stress disorder, psoriasis, schizophrenia, sleep apnea, tinnitus and Tourette's syndrome.

These studies impact policy in Israel and beyond. "When the science is done in Israel, it also filters outside," says Kaye.

For example, in early 2019, after Israeli researchers published results of a trial using medical cannabis for symptoms associated with autism spectrum disorder—more than 80 percent of the parents reported significant or moderate improvement in their child—three American states added autism as a qualifying condition for their medical-cannabis programs.

When government officials in nations from South America to Africa consult with iCAN, says Kaye, they learn that they don't have to do the research because they can rely on Israeli trials, which follow FDA-like protocols. Israel's

A prescription-carrying patient purchases medical marijuana at an Israeli medical-cannabis dispensary.

149

burgeoning medical-cannabis business landscape includes about 100 companies that grow, process and market strains for therapeutic purposes; develop technologies for cultivation or patient use; or develop pharmaceuticals for humans and pets. Kaye says the government is currently fielding more than 1,000 applications from would-be cannabis entrepreneurs.

"It's a rich environment in Israel because regulations make it easy to access the plant, and the government is putting money behind it from the Israel Innovation Authority," Kaye points out. In coming years, he predicts Israeli cannabis research will broaden its focus considerably: "We've got a plant with more than 300 molecules—not only cannabinoids but also many other compounds, like terpenes and phenols, that have therapeutic potential—and we have to have a competitive way to grow and extract those molecules to study their potential. Plus, the fairly recent discovery of the ECS opens up many research avenues for how cannabis interacts with the human body."

$17B
The value of the current estimated worldwide market for cannabis.

■ New Areas of Research
Other relatively new areas of research in which Israel has taken the lead are optimizing cannabis cultivation for the medical market, and standardizing cannabis-derived pharmaceuticals so that each dose is identical in strength and composition. This trailblazing work has been happening for the past five years at the Agriculture Ministry's Volcani Center,

under the direction of senior research scientist Nirit Bernstein, PhD.

Her lab studies how cannabis plants respond to various cultivation and environmental conditions, determines best practices for every step of the growing process, and identifies the cannabinoids and terpenes most effective for treating specific ailments. Interestingly, almost all the medically useful compounds in cannabis come from the flowers of unfertilized female plants.

"In our breeding program, we are developing strains suitable for medical indications such as multiple sclerosis or diabetes, and for agricultural properties such as disease resistance, high yield or improved standardization of the pharmaceuticals," Bernstein says. "I'm also working on developing new cultivars of cannabis. Most of those used today contain high concentrations of THC, but are not optimized for CBD and other cannabinoids and terpenes."

■ On the Cutting Edge
That's not the only science taking place. Consider these other research innovations:

At Hebrew University School of Pharmacy's Multidisciplinary Center for Cannabinoid Research, headed by Yossi Tam, DMD, PhD, a team of 30 scientists is conducting research on cannabinoids, endocannabinoids and medical cannabis, focusing on cancer, pain, inflammation, stress management, immunity, metabolism, drug delivery and

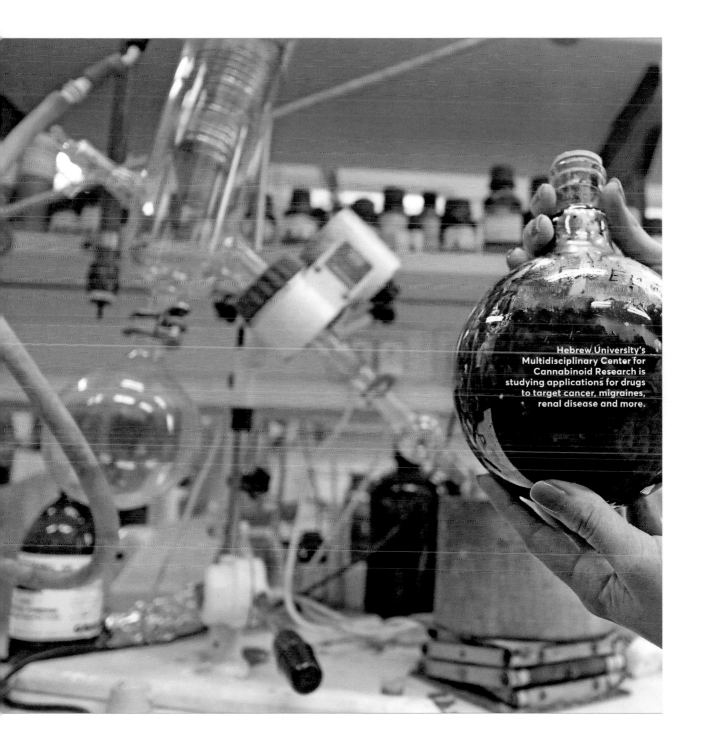

Hebrew University's Multidisciplinary Center for Cannabinoid Research is studying applications for drugs to target cancer, migraines, renal disease and more.

nanotechnology, pharmaceutical chemistry, neuroscience, plant science and genetics.

The Technion-Israel Institute of Technology's Laboratory of Cancer Biology and Cannabinoid Research, directed by David Meiri, PhD, investigates the therapeutic potential of cannabinoids for treating cancer, epilepsy and diabetes. The lab maintains databases of clinical data on cannabis patients, medical-cannabis usage in Israel and abroad, and cannabis strains used for clinical purposes.

Prof. Yosef Sarne at Tel Aviv University's Sackler Faculty of Medicine researches the ability of cannabinoids such as THC to protect the brain against age-related cognitive decline and neurodegenerative diseases including multiple sclerosis, Alzheimer's, Huntington's and Parkinson's diseases. Jerusalem-based Lumir Lab, headed by Prof. Lumír Ondřej Hanuš, has developed clinical validation and analytical methods to perform quality testing for the global medical-cannabis industry.

The Ben-Gurion University-Soroka Cannabis Clinical Research Institute in Beersheba recently published groundbreaking research on medical cannabis as a treatment for symptoms of autism, including seizures, tics, depression, restlessness and rage.

Lastly, Tikun Olam Research, a branch of Israel's largest medical-cannabis grower, performs clinical trials assessing proprietary strains and products in treating autism spectrum disorder, Crohn's disease, inflammation, Parkinson's disease, cerebral palsy, cancer, epilepsy and other conditions.

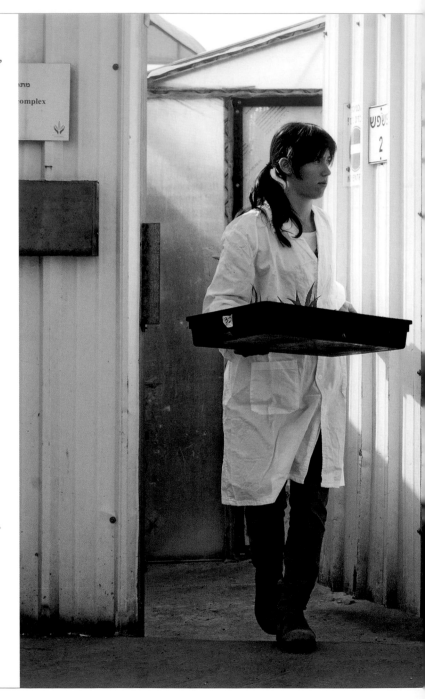

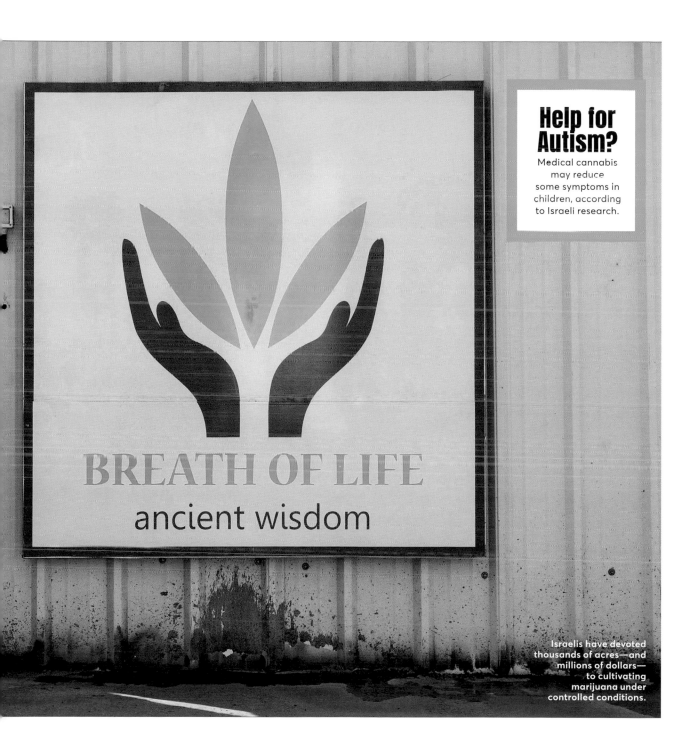

Help for Autism?

Medical cannabis may reduce some symptoms in children, according to Israeli research.

BREATH OF LIFE

ancient wisdom

Israelis have devoted thousands of acres—and millions of dollars—to cultivating marijuana under controlled conditions.

SPINNING A WINNING WEB

How seven brothers created the medication that changed how we see CBD.

Clockwise from top left: **1** Robert Werner helps with the Stanley brothers' high-CBD strain harvest. **2** The Stanleys' unique CBD strains have made Charlotte's Web world famous. **3** Jordan Stanley sorts through clones of his cannabis plants. **4** The Stanleys grow their cannabis on a 17-acre Colorado farm.

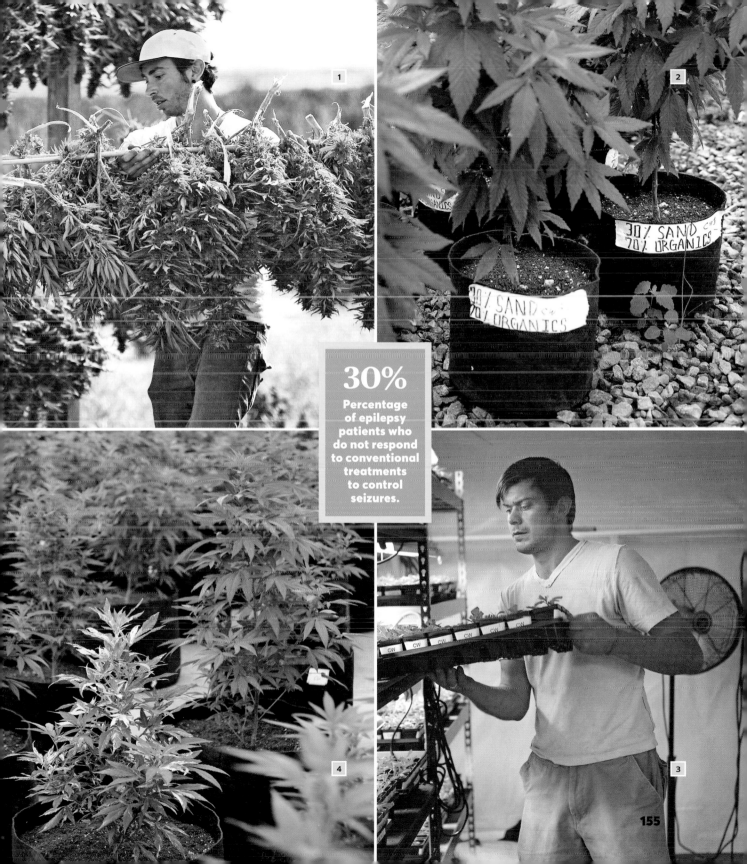

30%
Percentage of epilepsy patients who do not respond to conventional treatments to control seizures.

155

CBD CERTAINLY SEEMS HOTTER than a ghost chili these days. You can find it in everything from espresso shots to gummy bears to bath bombs to dog treats. Meanwhile, perhaps the most sizzling CBD company of all is Charlotte's Web (CWB), the top-ranked manufacturer and distributor of hemp-based cannabidiol medicines.

CWB ranks No. 1 in the world when it comes to hemp-based CBD sales. In 2018, for instance, CWB raised almost $100 million in an initial public offering (IPO) on the Canadian Stock Exchange (where both medical and recreational cannabis are legal nationwide). Since that IPO, shares of the company are up almost 90 percent. That increase is set to shoot even higher now, thanks to the 2018 Farm Bill passed by Congress and signed by President Trump. The legislation exempts hemp from the list of federally illegal controlled substances, at least as long as the plant contains less than 0.3 percent THC. Given this turn of events, the hemp-derived CBD market–which took in $190 million in 2018–is expected to grow to $22 billion by 2022. CWB stands to be a big part of that increase.

■ A Family Affair

The future looks green for the seven Stanley brothers, who started Charlotte's Web in 2013, but it's a far cry from their past. As kids, the siblings–Josh, Joel, Jesse, Jon, Jordan, Jared and J. Austin–grew up broke, first in small-town Oklahoma, then in Colorado. Always happy to make the best of a bad situation, though, whenever the family's electricity would get turned off, they'd just pull out candles and roast marshmallows to pass the time. When the boys wanted anything special, they knew they had to earn the cash themselves, so they'd take on odd jobs, like paper routes and candy sales.

■ Growing Their Business

It's this spirit of entrepreneurship that led the Stanley boys to dive into the world of medical marijuana in 2008, when their "uncle" (actually their mom's cousin) was diagnosed with pancreatic cancer. They helped him find cannabis-based treatments for his pain and discomfort, and were amazed by the improvements in his condition. Josh was the first to turn this discovery into a business opportunity. He'd broken his back so, like his uncle, he tried CBD treatments to help kick his dependence on the opiates he used for pain. He became such a believer that he opened Denver's Peace and Medicine Center, one of the city's first medical marijuana dispensaries. That same year, he called a family meeting to educate his mom and brothers about the business.

They wanted in. In 2009, Joel, Jesse, Jon, Jared and Jordan created the first two medical cannabis cultivation facilities in Colorado and started making oils to sell in the state's dispensaries. Two years later, Josh sold his dispensary and joined forces with his brothers. Their mission: to breed a strain of cannabis that was free of the intoxicating compound THC but

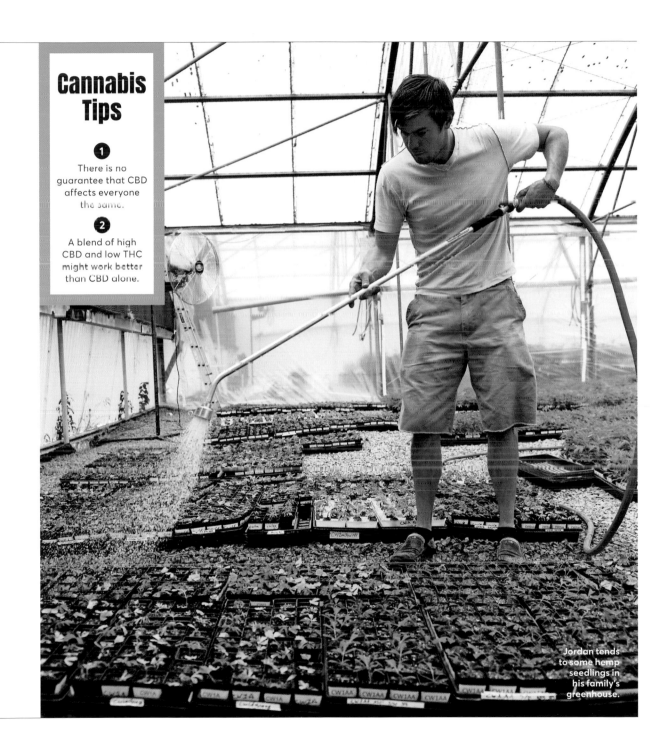

Cannabis Tips

1
There is no guarantee that CBD affects everyone the same.

2
A blend of high CBD and low THC might work better than CBD alone.

Jordan tends to some hemp seedlings in his family's greenhouse.

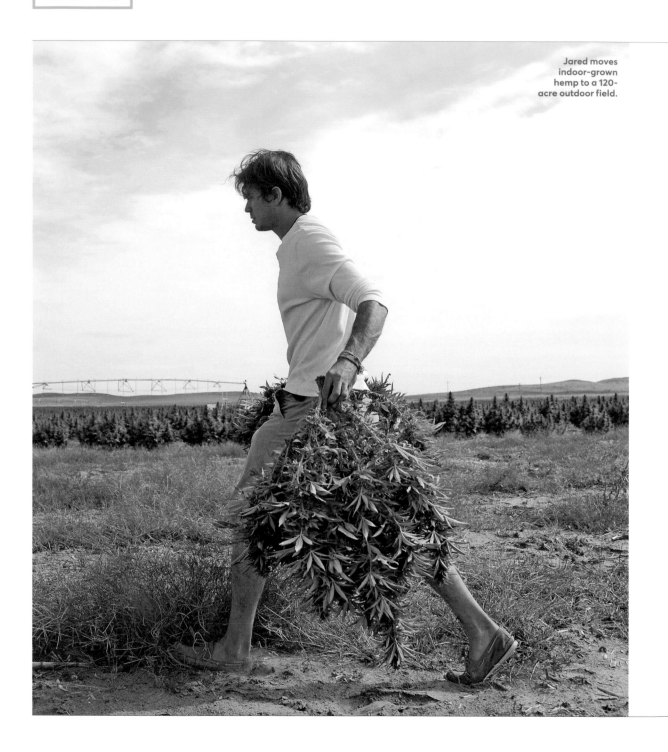

Jared moves indoor-grown hemp to a 120-acre outdoor field.

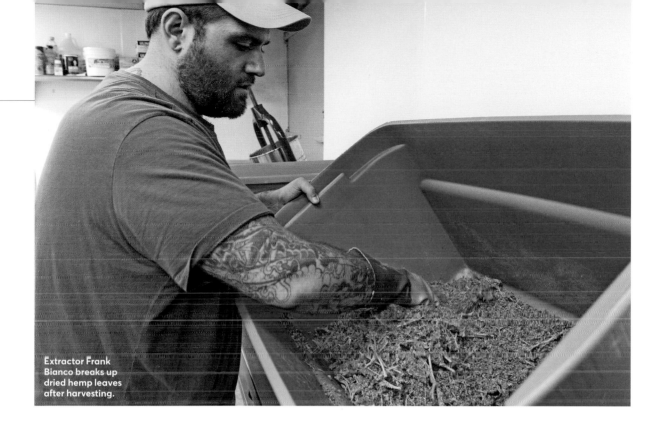

Extractor Frank Bianco breaks up dried hemp leaves after harvesting.

high in the nonintoxicating compound CBD. They succeeded, creating a strain they affectionately called Hippies' Disappointment because it was a plant designed to heal, not get you high.

As it turned out, their creation was anything but a downer. In fact, for one little girl named Charlotte Figi, it was a savior. By 2012, the then-5-year-old Charlotte, who had a form of epilepsy called Dravet syndrome, was experiencing hundreds of seizures a week. Her parents were desperate for something to control them, but were having no luck trying traditional medicine.

After some intensive research, they discovered that cannabis could be used to help. As good as that news was, they were concerned because they didn't want to get Charlotte high. That's when they heard about the Stanleys' low THC/high CBD weed and reached out to see if the brothers could create a similar extract that might help their little girl.

"When [Charlotte's mom] Paige called and told us about her condition, we were ready to help, until we learned Charlotte was 5 years old," Josh recounted in a TED/X lecture. However, after getting approval from Charlotte's doctors, the brothers got over their reservations and developed a nonintoxicating pediatric tincture. Almost immediately after the Figis gave Charlotte the medicine, their daughter went from hundreds of seizures a week to only one. So, in honor of this young girl, Hippies' Disappointment was rechristened Charlotte's Web.

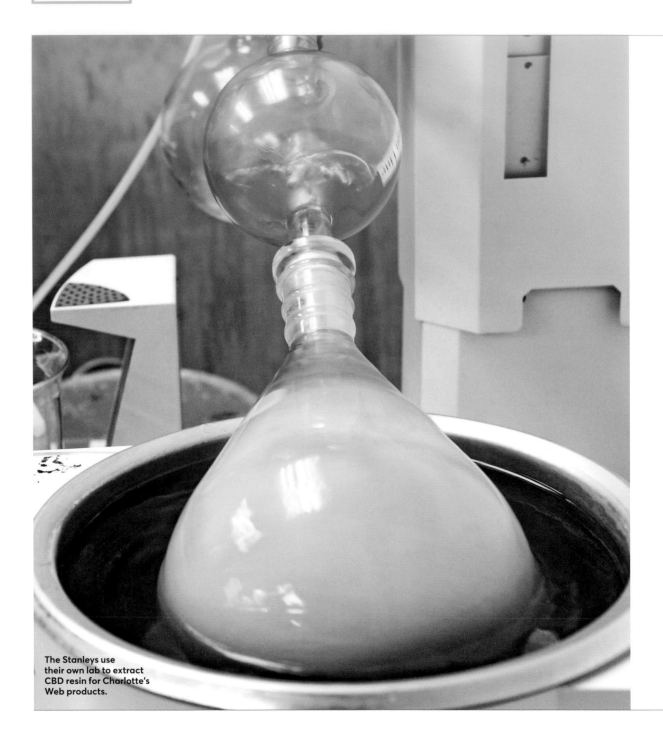

The Stanleys use their own lab to extract CBD resin for Charlotte's Web products.

■ Documenting Their Success

News of Charlotte's improvement reached CNN's Dr. Sanjay Gupta, and he included her in his groundbreaking 2013 documentary, *Weed*. While researching the documentary, which included interviews with the Stanley brothers and Charlotte, longtime cannabis critic Gupta actually changed his view of medical marijuana and became one of its most vocal advocates.

Joel Stanley credits Gupta's documentary for the increased national interest in the healing powers of CBD. Before *Weed*, he once explained in an Associated Press interview, "there was almost nothing with CBD in it. Very few people could even pronounce cannabidiol."

After his experience with Charlotte and the Stanleys, Gupta continued to explore the effectiveness of CBD treatments and eventually wrote, "I have seen more patients like Charlotte firsthand, spent time with them and come to the realization that it is irresponsible not to provide the best care we can as a medical community, care that could involve marijuana. We have been terribly and systematically misled for nearly 70 years in the United States and I apologize for my own role in that."

Once Gupta's documentary aired, the CBD stampede was officially on. It brought a sense of legitimacy to the idea of CBD as medicine and started a national conversation on the topic. Within months, there was a waitlist for

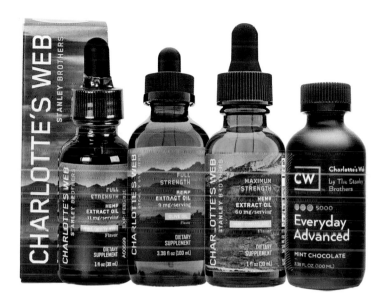

Charlotte's Web products are available as oils, isolates, capsules and topicals.

CWB's products, which now include vape cartridges and concentrate syringes as well as tinctures. Meanwhile, for patients hoping to learn about medical cannabis and CBD, the brothers founded Realm of Caring, a nonprofit that provides research, education and community for those using, or in need of more information about, medical marijuana.

Six years and one IPO later, what began as a family business is helping families around the globe. And while they've found financial success in cannabis, the Stanleys insist they are just happy to be helping. "We started this before there were any dollar signs," Joel told the AP. "We really believe in what we do, and our money is where our mouth is."

OPPORTUNITY KNOX

An Oregon family of doctors has a pioneering practice that advises patients on cannabis consumption.

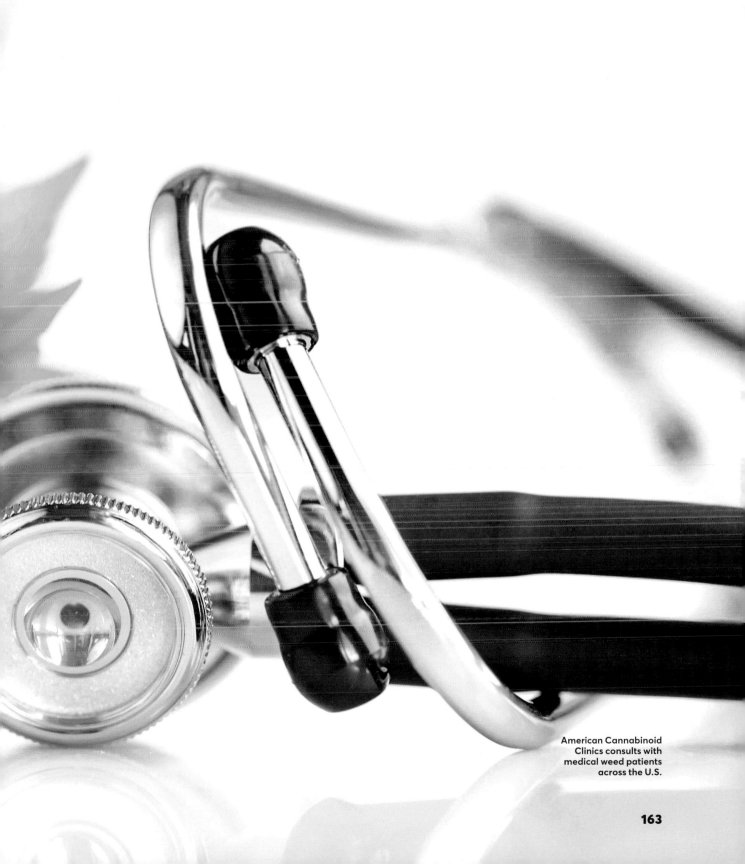

American Cannabinoid
Clinics consults with
medical weed patients
across the U.S.

MOST FAMILIES EVENTUALLY come up with some way for everyone in the clan to bond. For some, it's an ocean cruise. For others, it's an annual picnic. For still others, it's a simple trip to the cineplex or mall. For the Knoxes, however, it's all about the cannabis.

Husband-and-wife team Drs. David and Janice Knox have launched the Oregon-based American Cannabinoid Clinics, along with their daughters, Drs. Rachel and Jessica Knox. Their practice has offered what they call "integrative endocannabinoid medicine" since 2015, which means they consult with patients about how endocannabinoid medicine can help whatever ails them. The science of CBD is still relatively new, making it difficult to find doctors schooled in the ways of cannabinoids. So the ACC is definitely ahead of the curve when it comes to combining traditional medicine with cannabis-related healing.

"This is a family effort to answer the obvious needs of patients who see cannabis as an alternative to conventional medicine," explains Dr. Janice. "My family and I started out in the traditional medical-card-writing clinics, where it was obvious the patients needed more than the 10 minutes doctors were allowed to spend with them. These patients were looking for health-care providers who help with the safe use of medical marijuana for their many medical problems without being judged. We felt that we could answer this need."

We spoke with her to learn more about the services American Cannabinoid Clinics can provide, and how working in the cannabis field isn't just helping other families—it's also bringing hers closer together.

■ Has CBD been something your family has incorporated into your practice?
Yes. We practice cannabinoid medicine. We try to use the most appropriate cannabinoid for the medical condition to be addressed. CBD is the new "buzzword" cannabinoid. So this is a great cannabinoid to start most patients off with.

■ Among the four of you, do you each have a different expertise you bring to cannabinoid medicine?
Dr. David, an emergency room physician, is very scientific in his thinking and brings that perspective. Dr. Rachel, who is in family practice medicine, is not only knowledgeable in the science, but is also the chair of the Oregon Cannabis Commission. She is very involved in policy and regulations concerning medical cannabis in Oregon, and we all hope to influence regulation across the nation. Dr. Jessica is in preventative medicine and very knowledgeable in the science and does a great job on the speaking circuit, helping to establish endocannabinology as a discipline. I am in anesthesiology and love doing the research and thinking about possible formulations that will lead to safer and more efficacious medical therapies.

When you talk to your patients, what is the most common misconception they have about CBD and cannabis?

Most come in ready to use the products. However, they're looking for ways to take control of their health, and the propaganda about the harms of cannabis still lingers. They're concerned with getting high, needing to smoke and becoming addicted.

What separates ACC from others in the medical marijuana field?

I don't feel there are others out there doing what we're doing. Our goal is to help others understand that it's the physiology and lifestyle medicine that we are trying to address. It's not just about cannabis. It's about treating medical problems at the root cause and not just the symptoms. If we think and teach holistically, we're treating more than the symptoms of disease.

What are your top three tips for someone seeking to improve their health with CBD?

First, CBD is a great tool—but it needs help. Look to your food and nutrition for your first medicine. Second, look for safe, lab-tested and well-labeled products. Not all CBD product offerings are safe. And don't be afraid of using a ration that has some THC. Third, don't be afraid to adjust the dosage. Start low and go slow to titrate to symptomatic relief. The safety margin is wide.

You are based in Oregon, but if somebody lives in a different (and legal) state, can they still use your services?

We see patients nationally and globally by using our HIPAA-compliant telemedicine platform. They can either call our office or self-schedule at our website [theacclinics.com].

What effect has starting up American Cannabinoid Clinics had on the Knox family?

It's been fantastic. We've always been a close family. The joy of working together in this amazing space is beyond my dreams. The reactions we get from our colleagues, patients and the entire industry are very supportive and encouraging. I think we're a bit of an oddity to everyone, but it's fun.

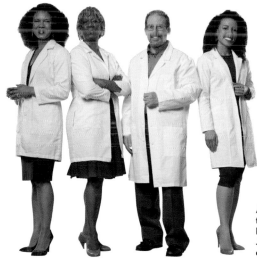

ACC is run by the Knoxes (from left): Jessica, Janice, David and Rachel.

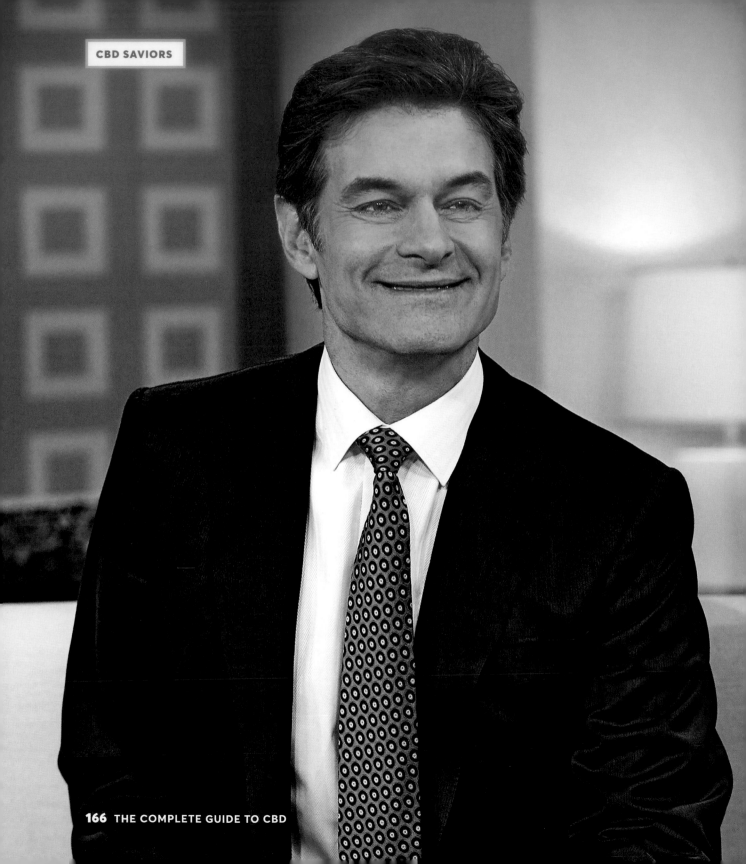

HE'S A BELIEVER

Beloved television personality Mehmet Oz is one of the world's most visible champions of medical marijuana. Just don't ask him to inhale.

DR. MEHMET OZ IS AN absolute buzz-master when it comes to manipulating the cycles of social media and tabloid television. He swears, however, that he's never copped a buzz.

"Just to be clear, I've never smoked a joint in my life," he tells me, in the clipped tones that have mesmerized his many fans. "I've never gotten high. I'm not an advocate of marijuana for recreational reasons, but I think that the evidence supporting the medical benefits of marijuana is clear."

A Harvard-educated cardiothoracic surgeon, Oz's word carries tremendous influence. His popular television and online broadcasts have garnered multiple Emmy awards, reaching more than 2 million viewers with a single episode. In 2008, *Esquire* magazine named him one of the 75 most important people of the 21st century.

So in championing medical marijuana over the past few years, Oz has played a key role in the growing acceptance of cannabis across America's vast heartland. He's even been able to spread the good word for weed in the Trump White House.

■ Cannabis Convert

The doctor's well-publicized belief in the plant's healing properties was inspired in part by the stories of his friends, such as billionaire sports entrepreneur Ed Snider.

"He developed a very bad bladder cancer and was dying," Oz tells me. "He was in terrible pain. The doctors were giving him opiates and opioids that wouldn't work—all the usual things you usually do for cancer patients. And this nurse said, 'I know you're a straight-up guy, but if you'd be willing to try just a little bit of marijuana, it might help take the edge off the pain. And maybe you won't be completely out of it on opiates.' So, he tried medical marijuana. It had a dramatic impact, and he lived a year without pain. His daughter, Lindy, has become one of medical marijuana's biggest advocates, and this is a blue-blood family from Philadelphia."

Pain and suffering are no respecters of the class system, and the TV doc found that elites were just as much in need of the healing powers of cannabis as some of the less well-heeled guests on his program.

"I hear stories like this over and over again," he says. "Like my close friend, Montel Williams. Here's a man who served his nation in the Navy, and then was told by that nation that his intractable multiple sclerosis pain could not be alleviated. Now he can't get out of bed without marijuana. He's become an advocate and has taught me a lot about it. He took me to dispensaries, and also where they grow the pot. Also, I've had guests on my show with children who have had seizures and experienced a complete remission of symptoms, thanks to medical marijuana."

The doctor has been particularly vocal about the efficacy of cannabis as an alternative to opioid drugs such as fentanyl for pain relief. "Medical

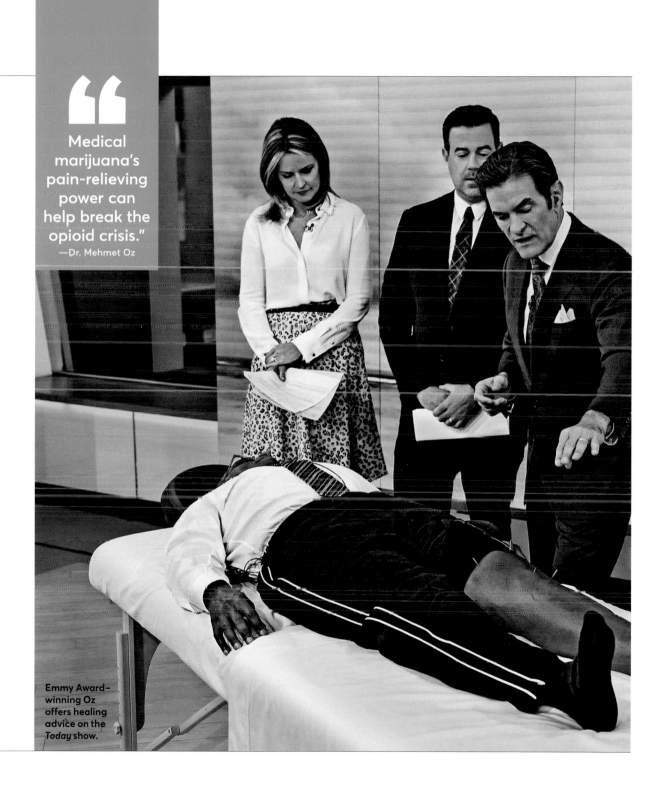

> **Medical marijuana's pain-relieving power can help break the opioid crisis."**
> —Dr. Mehmet Oz

Emmy Award–winning Oz offers healing advice on the *Today* show.

169

marijuana's pain-relieving power can help break the opioid crisis," he states. "I realized there's been a massive fraud in pain treatment. There was so much money being made using opioids to treat pain that there was almost a purposeful silence about other options. Nobody would research meditation, physical activity and things like medical marijuana for pain management."

■ Cannabis Needs to Be Medicine

The Dr. Oz Show has done much to fuel the CBD mania. But his personal response to the phenomenon is more muted. "I'm encouraged by it," he says, "but it's basically a work-around. CBD can be harvested from hemp, which is grown legally. But CBD is often more effective when there's a little bit of THC in the product. And that can only come from the marijuana plant. The terpenes in marijuana are also important. This needs to be medicine. It should be declassified and regulated by the FDA with very clear definitions of what percentage of CBD, THC and terpenes are recommended for specific medical conditions. If you have a headache, use this. If you have insomnia, use that. I can't recommend marijuana without knowing which strains are effective. I can't just prescribe Blue Kush any more than I could prescribe a 2014 merlot for a certain medical condition."

In 2018, Donald Trump appointed Oz to the President's Council on Sports, Fitness & Nutrition. This allowed

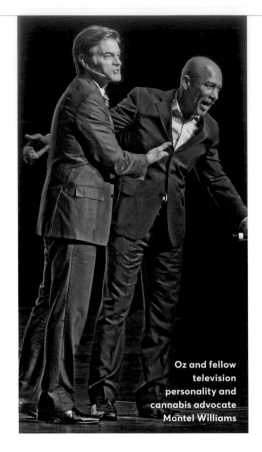

Oz and fellow television personality and cannabis advocate Montel Williams

the physician to speak with different agencies about declassifying cannabis as a Schedule 1 drug. "Nobody wants it to be Schedule 1," he said in a 2018 interview. "The FDA thinks it should be regulated. They don't think it should be Schedule 1. The DEA figures the DOJ [Department of Justice] doesn't want it around. Everyone is trying to figure everyone else out. Nobody wants to be on the hook for it. We need strong leadership that calls a spade a spade."

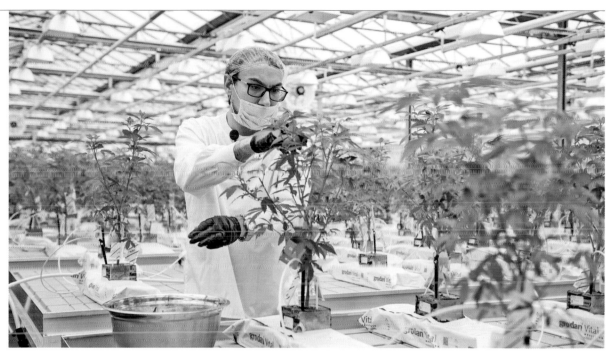

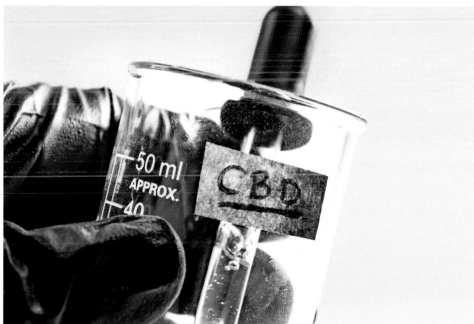

Above: A Canadian grow technician manicures a plant that is helping to put his country at the forefront of what could be a $150 billion-plus global market.
Left: CBD oil extract from cannabis flower

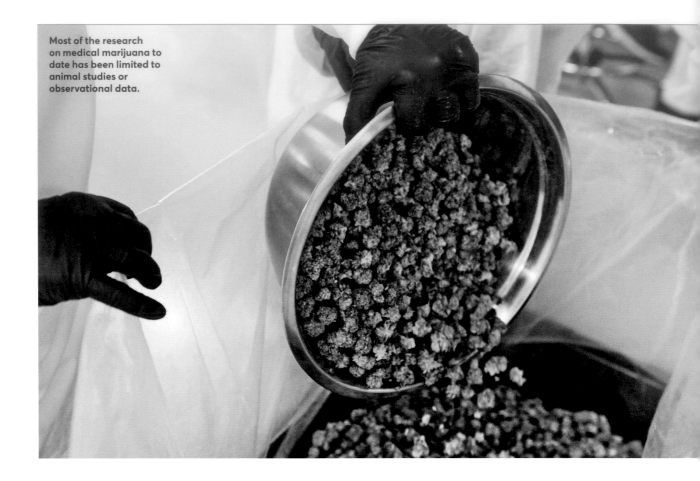

Most of the research on medical marijuana to date has been limited to animal studies or observational data.

■ Learning From His Viewers

Oz has already received a clearer directive from his millions of viewers and social media followers. Their support for cannabis legalization has been, he says, "overwhelmingly positive. There's a danger to society when people realize there's a law that's hypocritical. They stop following the law in general. An unfair law is very dangerous for a country. There may be a law that I don't like, but if I understand the rationale for it I can respect it. But if a country passes a law that has so little merit, it undermines all the laws that are fair. Where do you draw the line?"

Oz feels confident that Big Pharma—rather than Big Tobacco, major food and beverage companies and others who are now flocking to the cannabis space in large numbers—will eventually be the industry that will

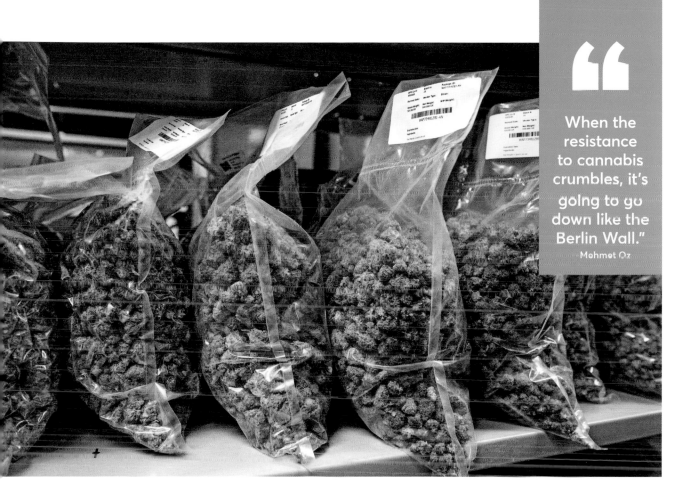

> ## "When the resistance to cannabis crumbles, it's going to go down like the Berlin Wall."
> —Mehmet Oz

come to control the lucrative marijuana marketplace.

"Pharma is already making inroads," he says, "and the smaller companies that are good are going to get bought. But unfortunately, American companies are way behind. Canadian companies are already producing products that will satisfy the huge U.S. demand, once our legal system catches up with the rest of the world. Most countries around the world won't allow marijuana, but the countries that are allowing the research—like Israel and Canada—they're going to be ahead. I think we need to move [cannabis] out of Schedule 1 and allow our researchers free reign."

Looking ahead, Oz predicts that cannabis change will be swift. "And when the resistance crumbles," he says, "it's going to go down like the Berlin Wall. It's ripe for a crash."

LEVELING THE PLAYING FIELD

A soccer star and her sister discover the benefits of using CBD for recovery and performance.

Twins Rachael (left) and Megan Rapinoe

The duo support each other on and off the field.

WHEN RACHAEL RAPINOE recounts her childhood, she frequently uses the word "we" to describe her time with her twin sister, soccer star Megan Rapinoe. "We grew up in Northern California, as part of a big conservative family. We focused on soccer and basketball. We ended up at the University of Portland playing soccer because we wanted to stay together–we dropped basketball due to height issues–and have had professional careers as athletes." At this point, Rachael and her sister Megan's paths diverged–and Rachael switches to "I." She recalls: "But I was riddled with injuries. I reached my physical capacity in training and recovery." While both sisters were making names for themselves around the world as elite soccer players, Rachael started to take opioids for pain and soon realized that she could no longer compete at the same level as Megan. "I was never mentally addicted, but I went through withdrawals and detox from opioids because I found that while I was on them, I never fully recovered."

Next Steps

As Megan's career took off, Rachael retired at age 26 and began to find her own path. She got a master's degree in exercise science, built up a strength-training and conditioning business, and coached. "My passion is the human body and keeping people at their best selves, both mentally and physically." Throw in an e-commerce business selling fitness apparel, and Rachael found a way to keep a foot in the sports world while establishing herself as an entrepreneur.

Then she met Kendra Freeman and Britt Price. "They were cannabis farmers in southern Oregon and kept telling me that CBD was going to be the future," Rachael recalls. "I kind of shrugged it off. Then cannabis became legal."

In Your Own Backyard

Suddenly, Rachael started to notice that many of the professional athletes she knew were using CBD as a recovery aid. "My network used cannabis products for recovery and also for sleep and relaxation, pre- and post-workout and games. I saw it in the locker room, with team doctors and physical therapists and even massage therapists. For me, this was a shift in perception. I wasn't used to people using cannabis and not getting high." The athletes she knew mostly used a high CBD/low THC strain, so she circled back to Kendra and Britt for more details.

The three decided there was a need in the industry for high-quality CBD products marketed specifically to female athletes of all skill levels.

"'Let's do this,' I recall saying to Kendra and Britt," says Rachael. And then things got real–fast. "Amy Margolis from The Initiative [an accelerator program for female cannabis entrepreneurs] knew Kendra and Britt, and the next thing I know, I'm sitting in my car in a parking lot before coaching a football game, trying to figure out a name for the company."

The team settled on Mendi, playing on the word mend, in hopes that it becomes its own verb or adjective. While the initiative felt intimidating, Rachael looked at it as an opportunity to define and sharpen her skills. "Since I am the CEO, the face of the company, I knew I needed help preparing and learning how to have cannabis conversations. I am an athlete; I loved the challenge." These newfound skills led to an impressive advisory board and financing. The team placed in the top 10 at Techfest (a demo fair for start-up companies), even without any product. "We had great exposure before anything else," adds Rachael, "so now it was time to keep up with the hype."

What happened next was a whirlwind of focus groups, feedback and fine-tuning to create a suite of three CBD products: a salve, gel capsules and gummies. That was followed first by a soft launch, then an actual launch and a variety of networking efforts.

Rachael says she knew she'd really made it in the cannabis industry when Mendi's credit card processor "experienced some issues with payments for over a week"–an event she considers a rite of passage.

■ The Future

Today, Rachael and Megan are back together. Megan is a board adviser, strategic partner and ambassador, providing athletes with product. "Athletes have an influential and strong voice that transcends CBD and even sports," Rachael says. "We want them to get behind Mendi and spread the word to their networks."

Rachael is connecting to people, from weekend warriors to full-time adventurers, as well as anyone searching for life balance to stay in top shape. "It is about a healthier solution to free people from distractions like pain, anxiety and insomnia," she says. This translates to a broader community, beyond professional athletes.

There are three things that need to happen before someone can appreciate the plant, says Rachael. "You have to see people that you trust use it. You have to try it for yourself and discover its efficacy. And finally, you have to hang out with other people in the industry." When the Rapinoes brought their mom to a party, her feedback was positive: "These are normal people trying to do good. Not drug lords."

Left: Mendi's hemp-derived gummies; right: the company's mantra

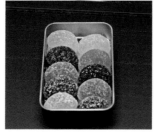
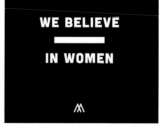

MILES AHEAD

Mile High Labs might be the most important cannabinoid company that you've never even heard of.

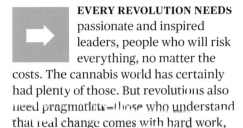

EVERY REVOLUTION NEEDS passionate and inspired leaders, people who will risk everything, no matter the costs. The cannabis world has certainly had plenty of those. But revolutions also need pragmatists—those who understand that real change comes with hard work, planning and attention to detail.

Stephen Mueller, founder and CEO of Mile High Labs, the preeminent global supplier of CBD ingredients, is one of those special leaders: a practical revolutionary with clear goals and a plan to reach them.

"We want to be the manufacturing backbone of the cannabis industry," Mueller states. "We want to be the largest and best at extracting and purifying ingredients from the hemp plant and manufacturing those ingredients into reliable finished products." That may not sound particularly sexy, but it's desperately needed.

Before he started Mile High, Mueller worked as an electrical engineer for clients like Apple, Purdue University and Raytheon. His job was to make accurate measurements for technology projects like the iPhone and missile-guidance systems. He brought this laser-like focus to the world of hemp-derived cannabinoids, and in three short years he has turned his company into the largest manufacturer of CBD isolate in the world. Mueller now oversees a 400,000-square-foot pharmaceutical production facility in Broomfield, Colorado.

We caught up with the engineer to talk about Mile High, his innovative, industrial-scale CBD extraction technology, his thoughts on the future of CBD regulation, and where he sees the industry heading.

◼ You were a successful engineer for some of the world's biggest companies. Why shift to CBD?

My background is in physics and engineering, and I wanted to get involved in a high-growth industry. I was interested in cannabis and suspected the CBD industry was going to get really big. I saw that you could grow as much hemp as you wanted without a lot of regulation from the state, and that there was a demand for CBD all over the world. You had this potentially large hemp supply, and you had this global market and demand for CBD.

But the problem was you needed some way to efficiently turn all that hemp into high-quality CBD. It was a problem nobody was really looking at. There were people doing smaller-scale extractions and purification, but nothing on the scale that I thought was going to be needed. As an engineer, it was a place [where] I thought I could add a lot of value and have a chance at having a successful business.

◼ There is a growing obsession with CBD quality and purity. Are there any real dangers to the consumer?

Yes. There are companies out there putting out inferior products. For example, our studies show that many of the products that claimed to have 1000 milligrams of CBD had nowhere near that amount–or too much.

Some had heavy metals, pesticides or microbial contamination.

A big part of our business plan is to put an end to all of that unethical production. Our ingredients are all audited. We're registered with the FDA, we're compliant with cGMP [current Good Manufacturing Practice], and we're one of the first ISO 9001-certified cannabinoid extractors. You can come and look at our facility; we're doing things the right way. So when we supply a company with CBD, their customers can be confident that their products were made in a compliant facility.

We're making investments in quality control that aren't necessarily appreciated, but we believe it's the right thing to do and it's the best thing for the industry. It will matter in the long term, from a business perspective.

The FDA has defined exactly how to produce quality ingredients, food products and medicine. It's really about implementing those established manufacturing practices. It adds more work and expense, but it's important to the long-term health of the industry to abide by the rules. About 20 percent of our company [employees] work in the quality-control department. I would suspect that's one of the highest percentages in the industry.

But until the FDA approves CBD, creates a regulatory pathway and starts enforcing it, you can kinda do whatever you want. And there are many who are cutting corners and doing things

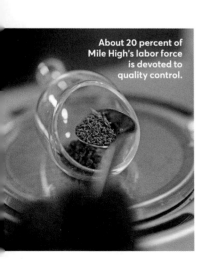

About 20 percent of Mile High's labor force is devoted to quality control.

as cheaply as possible. Honestly, some companies just don't know what they're supposed to be doing, and they don't care. Because the FDA has not yet recognized the legitimacy of CBD, you are forced to regulate yourself.

The FDA is in a challenging situation. It's not as if the government gets together and rolls out their initiatives in a coordinated way! You had the original Farm Bill in 2014, then another Farm Bill in 2018, and now the FDA has to figure out what they're going to do. You end up with some gray areas and it's a bit of a painful process.

But that slow evolution has allowed entrepreneurs, like Mile High, a chance to compete. We've had this period of time where the legality of hemp hasn't been so clear-cut, which tended to scare off bigger companies who couldn't handle the ambiguity. That allowed us to actually build something before we got squashed by whomever. The ambiguity has been a great thing for us!

■ **Tell us about the Mile High Monster.**
The Mile High Monster is the culmination of about two-and-a-half years of work, research and development. It's really what I've been working on since day one. I wanted to build something that was scalable and efficient for extracting CBD oil from hemp, and that's what this machine does. It will allow us to keep up with the demands of any Fortune 500 companies that will eventually want to buy CBD from us.

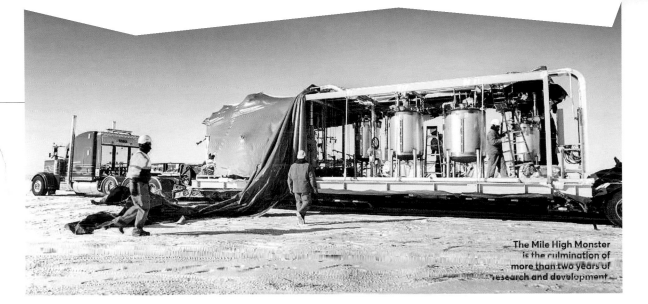
The Mile High Monster is the culmination of more than two years of research and development.

I sat down and started by designing a small-scale pilot plant, which allowed us to experiment and try out ideas without losing a lot of money. We solved hundreds of problems, which allowed us to efficiently build machines on a much larger, industrial scale. The Mile High Monster is the first piece of equipment of its kind specifically designed and built for processing industrial hemp. We were lucky to have the vision to see where the CBD business was heading a few years ago, because building the Monster was two solid years of work.

Did you accomplish your goal, or is there more development in the future?

There's definitely a lot more development that needs to be done. As far as extracting the crude oil, our machines do a fantastic job, but the industry and the technology are expanding so rapidly, I would never say, "We nailed it...it's time to kick our feet up." It's always about the next process and the next product. It's easier now because we have over 200 employees, including a bunch of chemists and engineers who are way smarter than me. We have a couple of new focuses. One is creating new extraction techniques that are more cost-effective and more efficient, and we're also looking at extracting other hemp compounds. I think the next two big cannabinoids are CBG [cannabigerol] and CBN [cannabinol]—especially CBG. I think we'll see a huge growth in that.

You recently launched a water-soluble division. Do you think CBD beverages will be important?

I think beverages have good potential. There are a number of companies already doing interesting things in the beverage space, but there are also some very big companies, like Coke for example, that are just waiting for the FDA to clarify things. Those could be very large customers in the future. I mean, beverages are convenient. Right now, the biggest CBD product is a tincture, but what's up with that? I think a beverage is much more convenient. I believe beverages and pills will eventually end up with a bigger part of the market share.

CBD UNLEASHED

Pet owners are increasingly turning to cannabis to treat their ailing animals.

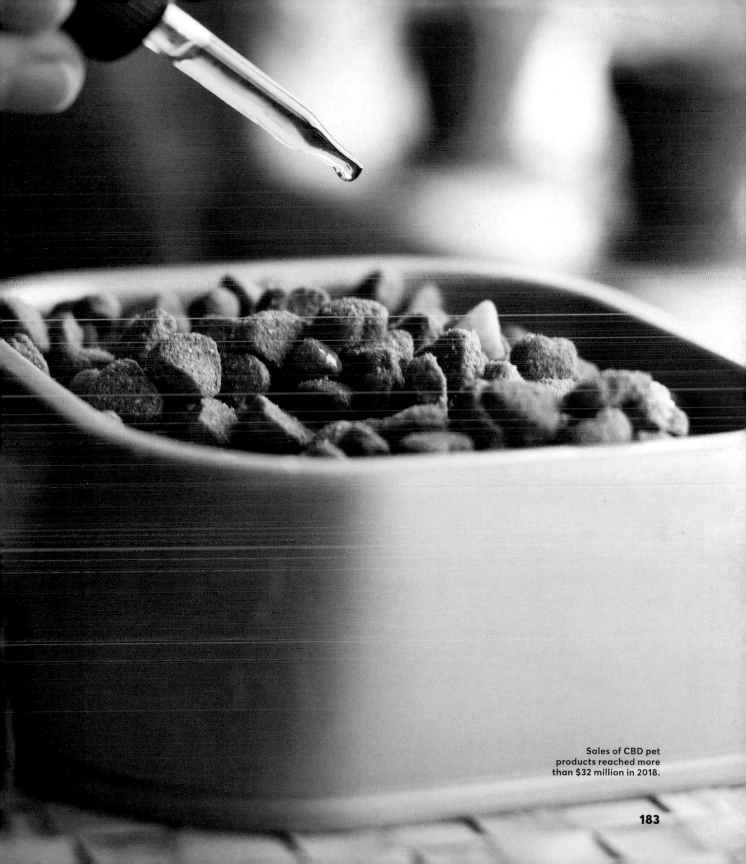

Sales of CBD pet products reached more than $32 million in 2018.

THE CURRENT HEALTH-CARE crisis isn't just affecting the human members of families across the country. It's also hitting the ones covered with fur pretty hard. According to the American Pet Products Association, people spent nearly $70 billion on medical treatments for their four-legged friends in 2017. With pet health-care costs expected to continue climbing, it's likely that dog and cat owners will keep turning to preventive treatments to help their animals. And, given its current popularity with people, it also makes sense that those treatments will include CBD.

According to Dr. Tim Shu, founder of VETCBD, which sells a variety of CBD products specifically formulated for household critters, cannabidiol can be effective for pets in the same way it benefits their humans. That's because people and their vertebrate cousins are born with the same endogenous cannabinoid system, which is made of both cell-produced endocannabinoids and cannabinoid receptors. CBD targets these receptors–located in the brain, organs, central nervous system and immune cells–to stimulate each body function's natural job, which is to promote healing, well-being and overall health.

Given this similarity between humans and animals, it's not surprising there seems to be nearly as many CBD-infused items for pets these days as there are for people. From vet-tested tinctures and oils to doggy treats, vitamin supplements, topical rubs and shampoos, hemp-derived products for animals are so popular that sales are expected to reach more than $125 million by 2022.

Despite this trend, organizations like the American Society for the Prevention of Cruelty to Animals have not yet endorsed CBD for pets. On its website, the ASPCA notes that "there are very few scientific studies looking at the efficacy and safety of CBD use in companion animals." Still, says an enthusiastic Shu, "It's an exciting time. Remember, the endocannabinoid system was only discovered in the 1990s and we're learning more and more every day. We're making strides in supporting everything like mood, memory, sleep, appetite and reproduction. The more we learn, the more our patients benefit, whether they walk on two legs or four. We're really just scratching the surface."

Shu and other animal experts are high on the use of CBD for several conditions, particularly these:

■ Seizures and Epilepsy
Roughly 5 percent of dogs in the U.S. suffer from seizures of one sort or another. While there's nothing conclusive as of yet, researchers believe high levels of CBD have shown promise in the management of your furry friend's seizures. Long-term therapy has indicated there's a reduction in frequency, and, in some cases, a complete elimination of them.

■ Canine and Feline Arthritis
As many pet owners have learned, larger cat and dog breeds are prone to arthritis.

Fortunately, CBD has been showing the same effectiveness in treatment for pets as it has for humans, since its anti-inflammatory properties target the inflammation of joints that causes the debilitating illness, as well as its accompanying pain. The good news for your pooch is that a landmark study conducted by a Cornell University-led team of researchers tested hemp-oil products on dogs and found that 80 percent of them saw significant decrease in pain and improved mobility.

Separation Anxiety

As is apparent in their faces when we say goodbye every morning, dogs are particularly prone to anxiety when their owners are away. Many pet owners use prescription medications to treat them, but according to two different independent reports, the two approved antidepressants for canine separation anxiety can produce vomiting and lethargy in between 45 and 85 percent of the animals that use it. CBD may be a safer option for this condition, as well as with the general anxiety that comes from traveling and hearing loud noises.

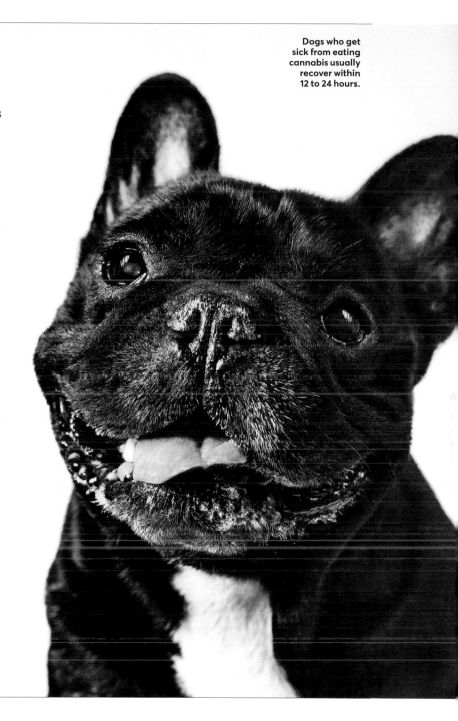

Dogs who get sick from eating cannabis usually recover within 12 to 24 hours.

SPECIAL THANKS TO CONTRIBUTING WRITERS
Jordana Benami, Tom Cunneff, Alan Di Perna, Nicola Farris, Elana Frankel, Sabrina Ford, Lisa Greissinger, Scottie Jeanette Madden, Natasha Swords, Brad Tolinski, Brooke Williams

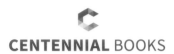

An Imprint of
Centennial Media, LLC
40 Worth St., 10th Floor
New York, NY 10013, U.S.A.

CENTENNIAL BOOKS is a trademark of Centennial Media, LLC

ISBN 978-1-951274-08-5

Distributed by
Simon & Schuster, Inc.
1230 Avenue of the Americas
New York, NY 10020, U.S.A.

For information about custom editions, special sales and premium and corporate purchases,
please contact Centennial Media at contact@centennialmedia.com.

Manufactured in China

Publishers & Co-Founders Ben Harris, Sebastian Raatz
Editorial Director Annabel Vered
Creative Director Jessica Power
Executive Editor Janet Giovanelli
Deputy Editor Alyssa Shaffer
Design Director Ben Margherita
Senior Art Director Laurene Chavez
Art Directors Natali Suasnavas, Joseph Ulatowski
Production Manager Paul Rodina
Production Assistant Alyssa Swiderski
Editorial Assistant Tiana Schippa
Sales & Marketing Jeremy Nurnberg